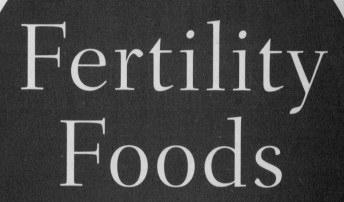

Fertility Foods

Optimize Ovulation and Conception Through Food Choices

JEREMY GROLL, M.D.

LORIE GROLL

A Fireside Book
Published by Simon & Schuster
NEW YORK   LONDON   TORONTO   SYDNEY

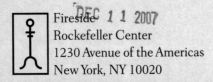 Fireside
Rockefeller Center
1230 Avenue of the Americas
New York, NY 10020

The names of some individuals in this book have been changed.

The views reflected in this book are not necessarily the views
of the United States Air Force.

For information regarding special discounts for bulk purchases,
please contact Simon & Schuster Special Sales at
1-800-456-6798 or business@simonandschuster.com.

Designed by Ruth Lee-Mui

Manufactured in the United States of America

10   9   8   7   6   5   4   3   2   1

Library of Congress Cataloging-in-Publication Data is available.

ISBN-13: 978-0-7432-7281-0
ISBN-10:   0-7432-7281-1

To our parents,
Monte and Karen Nowak, and
Marge and Jake Groll.
And to our children,
Libby, Michael, and Lainey.

You fill our lives with love and laughter.
You are our inspiration to help others
create their own families.
Thank you.

Contents

Introduction

MY NAME IS Jeremy Groll, and I'm a fertility doctor and research scientist. I've made it my life's work to help couples fulfill their dreams of having children. My wife, Lorie, and I are always thrilled when we find out that one of my patients has succeeded in conceiving a baby, and together, we came up with a way to stack the odds in our patients' favor. Then we realized—why not share it with the rest of the world? Why should our patients be the only ones with an unfair advantage? So we set out to write this book, which details all the advice and instruction you'd get from me if you came to my clinic.

Sure, we did it for the couples who were having trouble conceiving, but we had our own selfish reason, too: We live for this stuff. We want to get letters from couples all over the world, preferably accompanied by photos of their newborns. That's what will make our work worthwhile.

The "trick up our sleeve" is a diet and exercise program that will improve your insulin sensitivity and make you more fertile. It's a groundbreaking concept, and we've tested our methods over and over among my own patients and in clinical research. It works.

In this book you'll find all the instructions you need to maximize your fertility naturally, through simple changes to your diet and exercise routine. It's not a difficult diet program to follow, and you won't need lots of scales and calculators. We're even including a section of recipes to make your meal preparation as simple as possible.

We're also including chapters about vitamins and herbal supplements (which ones are good for you, and which ones are bad), what men can do to improve their fertility, myths about reproduction (Is there a "good" position for intercourse? Does it matter if men wear boxers or briefs?), ways to keep yourself on track, and support resources. If you want to understand all the science that goes into this program, there's a chapter about that, too—or you can choose to skip it and just follow the easy steps we provide.

You can try this program alone or in conjunction with other methods to boost your fertility to conceive. Even if you're already using medications or planning to undergo a clinical procedure, this program will improve your chances not only of conceiving, but of having a healthy, full pregnancy.

We're glad you've picked up this book, and hope you can soon count yourself among our success stories. We'll keep a space for your baby's photo on our office bulletin board.

Fertility Foods

One

The Starting Line

*i*MAGINE THAT YOU could fulfill your dream of having a baby just by changing the way you eat and making a few other lifestyle changes that won't cost you anything and might even be fun. Now imagine that I'm not kidding! The book you're holding in your hands right now could provide you with the least painful, least invasive, least risky way to get you from here to parenthood.

It's easy for most of us to accept that we can decrease our risk for problems like heart disease, diabetes, stroke, and cancer by eating right, exercising, and reducing stress. But some people believe that fertility is a game of chance—conception happens or doesn't happen, just on nature's whim. And when it doesn't happen, we sometimes turn immediately to expensive fertility treatments in a doctor's office because we assume that something is wrong with us and that we can't solve the problem on our own.

Let me say one thing up-front: I'm a fertility doctor, and by no means am I telling you that my profession is unnecessary. Indeed, I'm thankful to have helped countless women achieve healthy pregnancies when all the "natural" methods failed. But even expensive medical treatments are not foolproof; you can vastly increase your chances of conceiving by following the plan I'm about to share with you, whether you use it as your only fertility aid or in conjunction with medical treatment.

Lifestyle issues do indeed affect your reproductive health, in much the same way they affect your risk for heart attacks or strokes. Over the past few years, I've been perfecting a fertility program grounded in cutting-edge research and successfully used by the women who come to my clinic. Now that all the pieces of the puzzle are in place, I'm excited to present the program to you: I want to share my secrets with a wider audience so that my patients' success can be repeated by women all over the country. This is the first book of its kind; it's a balanced-nutrition diet and exercise program specifically designed for women who are trying to conceive.

The best news of all is that the lifestyle program I recommend can put you on track for better all-around health in addition to helping you achieve pregnancy and a healthy birth.

You're Not Alone

Problems with fertility seem to be on the rise in the United States. More than 9 million Americans of reproductive age are affected by infertility—men and women in about equal numbers—that is, at least one in every ten couples. And the number of visits to fertility specialists has skyrocketed in recent years; almost no other field of medicine has seen this kind of growth. But according to the American Fertility Association, only 5 to 10 percent of patients actually need high-tech procedures like in vitro fertilization.[1]

There are many causes of infertility, and you may find one or more factors that have contributed to your problem. The primary culprits are the following.

Age

Couples today tend to delay childbearing. First, they are getting married much later in life than couples in past years; the average age is now 27 for women and 29 for men, whereas it was 21 and 23, respectively, in 1970. More students than ever go to college and graduate school, and many women prefer to establish themselves in a career before having a baby. About 20 percent of women now wait until after age 35 to start trying to conceive, according to the American Society for Reproductive Medicine.[2]

Unfortunately, there's no getting around the fact that age is a major factor in fertility. Women are born with all the eggs they're ever going to produce; and over time, these eggs lose their quality and eventually the supply runs out. A woman's fertility starts to decline when she is in her late twenties, takes a stronger dip in her mid-thirties, and takes a severe downturn when she's about 39.

For men, age isn't as big a factor. Senator Strom Thurman was 81 when he fathered a child; and a 94-year-old currently holds the record for the oldest man to become a father.[3] However, according to a study published in the *Journal of Reproduction and Fertility* that compared men age 21 to 50 with men age 51 to 80, the latter group had 30 percent lower sperm production.[4] Sexual function in men also declines over the years, so it may be more difficult for men to achieve and maintain an erection. That can't be good for the chances of conceiving a baby!

Problems with Body Weight

Americans are getting fatter, and we all know it. From 1971 to 2000, the prevalence of obesity in the United States increased from 14.5 percent to 30.9 percent.[5] It's well documented that overweight and obese women have more reproductive problems than women in the normal weight range. Being overweight impairs ovulation, increases the risk of a miscarriage, and increases the risk of congenital defects. It also makes insulin resistance worse, and as you're about to learn, insulin resistance plays a major part in infertility. If your BMI (body mass index) is over 30, your fertility is definitely compromised. If your BMI is 28 or higher, weight is probably playing a role in your infertility.

On the opposite end of the spectrum, being underweight is a problem, too. You need at least 17 to 22 percent body fat to ovulate normally. Women who exercise excessively or whose bodies are deprived of proper nutrition tend to have irregular menstrual periods or no periods. This condition obviously has a poor effect on fertility.

The good news is that even a modest weight loss or gain, whichever is necessary, can greatly improve your chance not only of getting pregnant but also of having a healthy baby.

Pelvic Infections

You may have a sexually transmitted disease (STD) and never even know it. Chlamydia, for example, has surged in the United States and can be completely asymptomatic. It can also steal your fertility.

Four million new cases of chlamydia are expected this year, with some reports estimating that up to 20 percent of all sexually active female teenagers are infected. Most of them have no idea, and that is why chlamydia is often called the "silent STD." About 70 percent of chlamydial infections present no symptoms.[6] If symptoms do develop, they typically appear within three weeks of infection and may include genital discharge or bleeding, fever, genital itching, and abdominal pain. These symptoms are sometimes so mild and vague that women don't seek medical help, although at other times chlamydia results in full-blown pelvic inflammatory disease (PID), which may require hospitalization or surgery.

Gonorrhea has very similar symptoms, often exists alongside chlamydia, and can also harm fertility. About half of all cases of gonorrhea are asymptomatic, and an infected man is more likely to show symptoms than an infected woman.[7] Both of these diseases can be cured with antibiotics; but if they are not successfully treated, they can travel into a woman's fallopian tubes or a man's urethra and cause scarring and more serious infections.

Pelvic infections, which occur in the ovaries, fallopian tubes, and uterus, can usually be traced to STDs; but STDs are not necessarily the cause of such infections. Other possible culprits include gynecological surgery, insertion or removal of an intrauterine contraceptive device (IUD), and abortion. A recent study actually found that as many as 30 percent of upper genital infections are due to bacteria that are normally found in the vagina, thus resulting from no particular inciting factor.

Pelvic inflammatory disease is a severe form of pelvic infection. It's likely to start right after a woman's menstrual period and may cause abdominal tenderness, fever, and abnormal vaginal discharge and bleeding. The risk of infertility grows greater with each infection; it's estimated that a woman's risk of infertility is 11 percent after one PID episode, and then the risk doubles with each further episode. Women with PID are also 10 times more likely to have an ectopic pregnancy,[8] where the fertilized egg implants outside the uterus.

According to the Centers for Disease Control and Prevention (CDC), if not adequately treated, 20 to 40 percent of women infected with chlamydia and 10 to 40 percent of women infected with gonorrhea may develop PID.

What Do We Have to Gain?

Lifestyle changes can improve your "pregnancy forecast" in several ways: improved ovulation, decreased miscarriage, and lower likelihood of birth defects.

Right now, 10 percent of women who have regular menstrual periods have ovulatory problems. You'd never know it if your eggs were being released at the wrong time in your cycle, or if your eggs were damaged in some way. But both problems are often correctable with changes to your diet and daily routine.

The Insulin Crisis

A few years ago, my wife inadvertently changed my entire outlook on fertility. She and I were on vacation in Texas with our kids, and Lorie was venting about her inability to lose that last 10 pounds after the birth of our son. *Dr. Atkins' New Diet Revolution* and *Protein Power* topped the bestseller charts at the time, and Lorie was investigating the merits of these plans to figure out whether or not to try one of them.

As she described the science behind the plans to me, my eyes lit up. The plans were all based on improving insulin resistance, thereby decreasing insulin secretion, which allows for easier loss of fat—and easier pregnancy.

First, a few definitions are in order.

After you eat a meal, some of the food is converted into glucose, which is the simple sugar that provides energy to the cells in your body's organs. But your body doesn't use that glucose well unless your pancreas produces the hormone insulin. The insulin acts as a chaperone, helping your body deliver the glucose into your cells to use for energy. This keeps your blood sugar from getting too high.

The problem is that many people are insulin-resistant: their cells don't respond properly to the insulin. In turn, the pancreas tries to produce more and more insulin to compensate for the fact that not enough insulin is getting through to where it's supposed to go.

In time, the pancreas becomes unable to keep up. Eventually, extra glucose builds up in the bloodstream. This condition can lead to diabetes, a primary cause of heart disease, blindness, and nerve and kidney problems. The extra insulin stays in the bloodstream, too, promoting fat deposition, hindering fat breakdown, and causing a variety of metabolic effects that hinder fertility. This becomes a cycle, because extra fat makes it harder for muscles to process insulin, and that difficulty further adds to insulin resistance.

As you might suspect, we seem to be in an "insulin crisis" in this country. According to the CDC, the number of diagnosed cases of diabetes has risen 61 percent since 1991 and is expected to nearly double by the year 2030. The latest study by the World Health Organization (WHO) reports that 30.3 million Americans will have diabetes by then, compared with the 17.7 million who had it in 2000.[9] Of all the countries in the world, we have the third highest rate of diabetes both now and in future projections.

Some of the cause may be genetic, but this high rate is also a result of our lifestyle, including our diet. Recent studies conducted by Stanford University found that as many as 75 percent of Americans may be predisposed to developing insulin resistance. Normally, even if you have health conditions (such as diabetes, polycystic ovary syndrome, hypertension, or obesity) that make you a very likely candidate for insulin resistance, your doctor won't test you for insulin resistance, because it's very complicated to measure and diagnose. But our lifestyle choices can prevent this problem, just as people who are predisposed to alcoholism can stop the problem by never taking a drink.

Now, here's why Lorie's discussion sparked my excitement.

Insulin and Fertility

We took our vacation right after I had presented a lecture about much of the recent groundbreaking research on polycystic ovary syndrome (PCOS), a common problem that brings women to fertility clinics. The InterNational Council on Infertility Information Dissemination estimates that 5 to 10 percent of women have PCOS, but most of them haven't even heard of this disorder—at least until they visit fertility clinics trying to figure out why they can't conceive.

Most women with PCOS are overweight, and their symptoms may include excessive hair growth on the face or body, missed or irregular menstrual periods, acne, dandruff, skin tags, and dark patches of skin. Some women have all these symptoms, and some have none. Unfortunately, PCOS stops women from ovulating and often leads to infertility.

My lecture focused on how insulin resistance contributes to the syndrome. But even if you don't have PCOS, it's very possible that you have insulin resistance. High insulin levels stimulate the ovaries to overproduce the male hormone testosterone, which wreaks havoc on normal ovulation. I'm sure you can imagine what this means for fertility: if a woman isn't ovulating properly, her chances of conceiving a baby are slim.

As Lorie talked about the various diets meant to alleviate insulin resistance, I realized that it was possible for us to come up with a diet that would not only improve the way a woman's body uses insulin but, in so doing, also bring back her fertility!

That's when I began formulating my plan: a diet and exercise program meant specifically for women who are trying to conceive. I used concepts similar to other reduced-carbohydrate approaches, but I altered the programs to suit ovulatory function and women's reproductive needs in particular, on the basis of cutting-edge research. If you're already on a low-carb diet, you're probably already on the right path. We'll just tweak the diet a little, showing you what you can change and add to make it optimal for fertility.

What's more, you don't have to have a diagnosis of PCOS to benefit from this plan. PCOS led us to the connection between insulin and fertility, but whereas PCOS is found in 5 to 10 percent of women of reproductive age, as much as 75 percent of the population is prone to develop insulin resistance. This means that, for three out of four of us, insulin insensitivity is affecting our health to some degree. Regardless of the underlying problem hindering your fertility, in order to overcome it you must ensure the ability to produce a mature egg and to have the resulting embryo attach properly to the uterus. We will show you how adhering to our plan will optimize these processes and help achieve a successful pregnancy no matter what the obstacles may be in your own case.

First Success

It all started with Nicole. Once I had made the connection between an insulin-reducing diet and fertility, I needed to find out if the diet would be effective. Nicole was a 28-year-old woman who had been trying to conceive for two years. Her menstrual cycles were irregular, occurring every two or three months.

I spoke to her about my nutritional recommendations: a diet that would enable her to keep her insulin levels on an even keel and lose some weight. She lost eight pounds within two months, and achieved a successful pregnancy on the second cycle after starting the program.

We were on to something. I could barely contain my excitement as I congratulated Nicole. It was at this point that I knew we were going to help a lot of people, maybe even some people who had already tried all the usual infertility treatments and failed—people who thought they would never be able to have a child of their own. And we were going to do it in a way that was low-cost, painless, and free of detrimental side effects.

The Test

After a few more successes like Nicole's, I knew it was time to do a wider-scale randomized clinical trial. The Surgeon General's Office was excited about my idea, too, and gave me a $10,000 grant for a study to test the effectiveness of an easy-to-follow, balanced-carbohydrate weight-loss plan for infertile women.

In this clinical investigation, I enlisted a group of overweight, infertile women, of whom some had PCOS and some didn't. For six months (or until they achieved pregnancy), each woman either followed the standard diet recommended by the American Diabetes Association (ADA) (not low-carbohydrate) or my balanced-carbohydrate diet. All patients received individual counseling.

This study is ongoing, but the early results look wonderful. The women following my plan showed improved insulin resistance and ovulation, with a few pregnancies achieved, whereas the women on the ADA diet did not. Both groups lost a modest amount of weight.

Carbs and Insulin

Mine is not the only study to have tested how diet can affect insulin resistance.

A study reported in the medical journal *Metabolism* in 1994 found that a low-carbohydrate, high-protein diet helped insulin resistance, whereas a high-carbohydrate, low-protein diet made insulin resistance worse.[10]

Similarly, a study done in 1996 by the Department of Internal Medicine of University Hospital Geneva found that a diet containing 25 percent carbs improved insulin resistance, whereas a diet that included 45 percent carbs did not.[11]

Get to the Part Where I Have to Eat Hamburgers for Breakfast

O ye of little faith. I promise that nothing about our plan is extreme or radical. I don't believe that food groups were put on this earth to tease us into looking but not tasting, I don't believe you need to run marathons to stay healthy, and I don't think you should have to perform mathematical equations more complex than anything a calculus professor could dream up just to eat a proper meal.

In short, this revolutionary fertility plan is built to optimize your insulin secretion. To do that, you'll have to limit carbs, but not eliminate them. The key will be balancing protein and complex carbohydrates at each meal and snack to lower insulin stimulation. Starchy carbs must be curtailed as much as possible.

The second part of the food plan is timing. You're going to learn how to space your meals and snacks throughout the day, eating a total of five times a day. You'll have an early breakfast, lunch, a midday snack, dinner, and a nighttime snack. (Yes, you do get to snack at night!) Regularly timed meals and snacks stop your body from going into a fasting state, which slows down your metabolism.

Work It Out

There is also an exercise component to this plan. Getting your body moving also improves insulin response, so we'll make sure to get you on track for 30 minutes of exercise five times a week. The exercise will be divided between low-impact aerobic activity and resistance exercising.

Planning and Emotional Support

As you've probably experienced, when you're jazzed up about something—even something challenging—it isn't hard to get started. What can be difficult, however, is seeing the project through for more than a few days. That's why it's important to set specific goals for yourself, write them down, and find a source of emotional support.

Of course your overall goal is to get pregnant, but you can't control when that happens, so it's more important for you to set goals that you can directly control. You'll track your goals related to diet and exercise.

Keeping a journal is a proven way to help people achieve all kinds of goals, and later, it can serve as a memento—in this case, a memento of how dedicated you were to your child before he or she was even conceived. We'll also direct you to support groups in person and online. Having someone to check in with can make all the difference between just starting a plan and actually sticking with a plan. We all tend to be more disciplined when we feel accountable for our actions, and a friend, spouse, or support person can be the perfect motivator if the temptation to slack off creeps up.

Fertility Treatments: In Tandem or Solo

Many problems with fertility do require some sort of medical intervention, whether simple treatments or surgery. Some fertility problems, too, are associated with long-term medical risks. So it's important that if you're having trouble conceiving or carrying a pregnancy once you have conceived, you do get an evaluation by a reproductive endocrinologist.

Regardless of the cause of your infertility, though, all treatments will require proper maturation of an egg and attachment of an embryo to the uterus. The plan in this book will complement any fertility treatment plan by giving you an advantage in both of those areas, and in some cases it will make medical treatment unnecessary altogether. This is especially important for some people whose religious or moral beliefs prohibit them from utilizing some of the available reproductive technologies.

We know that fertility treatments can be expensive; and in writing this book, we hope to provide a way to cut down the expense. You may wind up needing fewer treatments or shorter care, or you may wind up never having to see the inside of a fertility clinic again. If you were one of my patients, though, please at least wave as you drive by my office!

Now let's get you started.

Two

The Food Guide

ﬁIRST, LET'S EASE your worries. This isn't a starvation diet, nor is it particularly limited or difficult to follow. Our nutritional program, formulated from the most recent science and clinical research, is designed to create an optimal environment in your body to help you achieve pregnancy, while satisfying your appetite and not driving you crazy in the process. Who needs extra stress when you're trying to conceive or maintain a pregnancy?

Although we're putting this food guide near the front of the book, please note that it is not the only step of this program. It's an important part, but the other components are also essential if you want to improve insulin resistance, optimize your ovulation, and see results.

Additionally, these recommendations are fairly specific for women and men of reproductive age. People's metabolism and nutritional requirements change throughout life. You may see other nutritional plans that differ in some aspects from this plan because they're meant for a broader target population. Everything in this plan is tailored specifically for your particular situation.

There is no "magic food" that will attract a baby to your womb. Believe me—I, too, wish I could tell you that three bars of Belgian chocolate a day would do the trick. But there are particular combinations of foods and nutrients that will help you, and other types of foods and supplements that can hurt you.

Our goal is to guide you to create your own menus, not to dictate the exact meals you must consume. We do provide a sample meal plan in Chapter 3, but our experience tells us that most people aren't thrilled about following a prescribed program that tells them they must eat cottage cheese at 7 a.m., an orange at 9 a.m., and so on.

You'll find specific guidelines here for the amount of certain nutrients you need and how to time your meals, but you get to decide what you eat. We'll teach you how to choose foods that appeal to you and that will help your body produce the optimum amount of insulin and other hormones to boost your fertility. When you learn the principles of composing fertility-enhancing meals, it will be much easier for you to create suitable meals if you're in a situation where the exact food items on our sample meal plans are not available. After reading this chapter, you should be able to put together an appropriate meal at home, in a restaurant, or just about anywhere else that you may find yourself.

Before we make recommendations, we'd like you to understand just why we're making them, so let's spend a little time understanding how our bodies use food, and how that process relates to fertility.

Crash Course on Nutrition

When we consume food, our bodies are looking for two things: macronutrients and micronutrients. Macronutrients are protein, carbohydrates, and fats; micronutrients are vitamins and minerals.

Protein

Proteins are made up of chains of chemicals called amino acids, which are essential for the growth and repair of nearly every structure in the body. A protein's nutritional value is calculated on the basis of how many types of amino acids are present and their overall quantity. Our bodies can make 13 types of amino acids—they're classified as nonessential amino acids because we don't need to get them from an outside source. There are nine amino acids known as essential amino acids, and the only way to get them is through protein in food. If a protein has all the essential amino acids, it's called a complete protein. If not, it's an incomplete protein.

Protein is the main component of our muscles, organs, and glands and is necessary for children's growth. Although the body's primary source of energy is carbohydrates, about 10 percent of our energy comes from protein.

Our bodies can't store essential proteins, so we need to get our minimum daily protein requirement from food every day.

Carbs

Carbohydrates are the body's main source of energy. After we eat a meal, the liver breaks down carbohydrates into glucose (blood sugar), which is absorbed into the blood and travels to the tissues to provide energy. The brain is the biggest glucose hog.

Carbs are also the primary insulin stimulators; as your blood glucose rises, your pancreas releases insulin to deal with it.

Think of glucose as kindling for a fire—little pieces of wood that burn easily when you light them. But like kindling, glucose gets used up quickly. To sustain a more constant source of energy, we need a storage system. Without such a system, we'd need to eat continuously, like little Pac-men and Pac-women, gobbling up all the carbohydrates in sight so that we wouldn't run out of energy and die.

Fortunately for us, our bodies do have storage systems in place. When we eat more carbs than are needed immediately for energy, the glucose is stored in a string of molecules called glycogen. The glycogen hangs out in two places: the muscles and the liver. The brain can't access the glycogen stored in the muscles. The limited amount that is stored in the liver can later be processed and sent back into the bloodstream to maintain the necessary level of blood sugar.

Those storage tanks in the muscles and liver, however, don't amount to much. Once our limit of glycogen is filled, the excess glucose gets converted into fatty-acid molecules and is stored in fat.

Fat

If we think of glucose as kindling, then we can think of fat as a log of wood. It contains a tremendous amount of energy, but if you put a match to it, it won't readily burn. It needs to be shaved down into little pieces, back into kindling, to catch fire. Fatty acids in fat tissue must be converted back into glucose to provide the body with energy.

Fat, despite what you may have heard, isn't an evil that must be eradicated. The body needs fatty acids. They're important for cell membranes, nerve function, and cellular communication, and as we've just mentioned, they can be stored for future energy needs.

And did you know that fatty acids are the "off" switch for your appetite? Researchers have discovered that when the body has digested the required amount of fatty acids, messages are sent to the brain to say that we're full. This is why you often remain hungry on a low-fat diet; there's nothing available to turn off your appetite switch!

Insolent Insulin

Although many details surrounding the hormonal control of glucose metabolism remain mysterious, the basic process isn't too hard to understand. Insulin acts as the "glucostat" to regulate your blood sugar after a meal. When the level of blood sugar is high, insulin drives it down by corralling excess glucose into storage for later energy needs. Once the level of blood sugar is in the optimal range, insulin secretion stops and allows the fat tissues to release their energy stores to meet the body's ongoing need for energy.

At least, that's the plan. But frequently, our glucostat goes haywire. When the body doesn't respond to insulin as well as it should, we develop insulin resistance. In this condition, the body secretes more and more insulin to keep glucose levels in check. When the insulin level stays high, the body remains in "storage mode" for prolonged periods, so that energy is encouraged to turn to fat, and fat breakdown is discouraged. You can think of insulin as a very anxious hormone prone to doomsday thinking. Insulin wants the body to store fat and keep it stored in case we ever face a desperate food shortage. Worst of all for our purposes, insulin also negatively affects a woman's fertility.

Studies have found that keeping insulin levels low helps a woman's reproductive function. That's the basis for this program, so we're going to make sure that what you eat gives you the best chance to reduce insulin resistance.

The Glycemic Index

You may be familiar with the concept of the glycemic index (GI) and glycemic load. These are measurements of the quality of carbohydrates. The GI compares and ranks foods according to their immediate effect on glucose levels, and the glycemic load measures the GI score multiplied by the amount of carbohydrates, divided by 100.

The GI and the glycemic load reflect traits such as the ease with which a food is digested, the amount of fiber it contains, and the type of sugars present. For example, foods containing fructose have a lower glycemic load because the body breaks down fructose fairly slowly. Carbs that break down quickly are likely to make blood sugar spike, whereas carbs that break down slowly release glucose on a more steady, prolonged basis, which doesn't tend to send insulin into a tizzy.

In this program, we ask you to avoid foods with a high glycemic load; that is, foods that send your blood sugar soaring and contribute to insulin resistance. Starchy and sugary foods are the worst culprits: pancakes, syrup, white potatoes, scones, and jam make up a portion of the list of foods to avoid.

The Insulin Index

What about foods that contain more than one type of nutrient? Dairy products, for example, contain fatty acids as well as some protein and carbs in the form of lactose. Because lactose is a sugar, it will trigger insulin to react to keep blood sugar levels in check. So how do you calculate the effects that foods like this have on insulin?

Luckily for us, researchers created the insulin index for just such a scenario: to measure the insulin response after a specific food is eaten. This scale is more helpful for assessing the insulin effect caused by the digestion of foods like meats, eggs, and cheese—foods that are not broken down into glucose. However, the insulin effect for these types of food tends to be much lower than the effect for carbs and will contribute only a small percentage of the insulin stimulus created by the meal as a whole.

According to Professor Jennie Brand-Miller, a leading authority on the glycemic and insulin indexes, the two indexes correspond closely to each other. On the basis of this information and the fact that the bulk of research has been conducted in terms of the glycemic index, we'll use the glycemic index as the reference point throughout this book, to keep the instructions as simple as possible.

If you do want to investigate the insulin index further to tighten your insulin control, research away! It can only help. Here are a couple of links to get you started:

- www.mendosa.com/insulin_index.htm
- www.zonehome.com/zlib0025.htm

Determining Your Nutritional Needs

To get an idea of your daily nutritional needs, check the table below. Look up your height in inches on the left, then trace over to the right to find your current daily protein, carbohydrate, and fat requirements in grams. Either highlight this information or write it down in the space provided in the worksheet on page 22. These numbers will soon become as familiar to you as your phone number and your social security number.

DAILY NUTRIENT REQUIREMENTS

Height	Daily Protein Requirement	Daily Carb Requirement	Daily Fat Requirement
5 feet, 0 inches (60")	82 grams (g)	82 g	20–25 g
5 feet, 1 inch (61")	83 g	83 g	21–26 g
5 feet, 2 inches (62")	88 g	88 g	22–27 g
5 feet, 3 inches (63")	90 g	90 g	23–28 g
5 feet, 4 inches (64")	92 g	92 g	23–29 g
5 feet, 5 inches (65")	95 g	95 g	24–30 g
5 feet, 6 inches (66")	96 g	96 g	24–31 g
5 feet, 7 inches (67")	97 g	97 g	24–31 g
5 feet, 8 inches (68")	100 g	100 g	25–32 g
5 feet, 9 inches (69")	101 g	101 g	25–33 g
5 feet, 10 inches (70")	102 g	102 g	26–33 g
5 feet, 11 inches (71")	104 g	104 g	26–34 g
6 feet, 0 inches (72")	105 g	105 g	27–34 g
6 feet, 1 inch (73")	106 g	106 g	27–35 g

The scientist in me wants to tell you that this is an extremely simplified way to determine your protein requirements; more precise calculations can be made by determining your height, waist circumference, and hip circumference, or by using special calipers to measure body fat. However, the practical side of me realizes that using the table we've just given is far simpler and is good enough for our purposes.

To make this table, we calculated the daily requirements for each height using a weight that gives a body mass index (BMI) of 29, which is around average for American women. If you know that your BMI is not in this range, or if you'd like a more precise measurement of your nutritional needs, follow these instructions:

1. Measure your hip circumference (to the nearest half-inch) at its widest point three times, then calculate the average.
2. Measure your waist (to the nearest half-inch) at the belly button three times and take the average.
3. Measure your height to the nearest half-inch.
4. Take those measurements and use this table to find the corresponding constants *A*, *B*, and *C*.

Hip		Abdomen		Height	
Inches	Constant *A*	Inches	Constant *B*	Inches	Constant *C*
30	33.48	20	14.22	55	33.52
30.5	33.83	20.5	14.40	55.5	33.67
31	34.87	21	14.93	56	34.13
31.5	35.22	21.5	15.11	56.5	34.28
32	36.27	22	15.64	57	34.74
32.5	36.62	22.5	15.82	57.5	34.89
33	37.67	23	16.35	58	35.35
33.5	38.02	23.5	16.53	58.5	35.50
34	39.06	24	17.06	59	35.96
34.5	39.41	24.5	17.24	59.5	36.11

35	40.46	25	17.78	60	36.57
35.5	40.81	25.5	17.96	60.5	36.72
36	41.86	26	18.49	61	37.18
36.5	42.21	26.5	18.67	61.5	37.33
37	43.25	27	19.20	62	37.79
37.5	43.60	27.5	19.38	62.5	37.94
38	44.65	28	19.91	63	38.40
38.5	45.32	28.5	20.27	63.5	38.70
39	46.05	29	20.62	64	39.01
39.5	46.40	29.5	20.80	64.5	39.16
40	47.44	30	21.33	65	39.62
40.5	47.79	30.5	21.51	65.5	39.77
41	48.84	31	22.04	66	40.23
41.5	49.19	31.5	22.22	66.5	40.65
42	50.24	32	22.75	67	40.84
42.5	50.59	32.5	22.93	67.5	40.99
43	51.64	33	23.46	68	41.45
43.5	51.99	33.5	23.64	68.5	41.60
44	53.03	34	24.18	69	42.06
44.5	53.41	34.5	24.36	69.5	42.21
45	54.53	35	24.89	70	42.67
45.5	54.86	35.5	25.07	70.5	42.82
46	55.83	36	25.60	71	43.28
46.5	56.18	36.5	25.78	71.5	43.43
47	57.22	37	26.31	72	43.89
47.5	57.57	37.5	26.49	72.5	44.04
48	58.62	38	27.02	73	44.50
48.5	58.97	38.5	27.20	73.5	44.65
49	60.02	39	27.73	74	45.11
49.5	60.37	39.5	27.91	74.5	45.26
50	61.42	40	28.44	75	45.72
50.5	61.77	40.5	28.62	75.5	45.87
51	62.81	41	29.15	76	46.32
51.5	63.16	41.5	29.33	———	———

(continued)

Hip		Abdomen		Height	
Inches	Constant A	Inches	Constant B	Inches	Constant C
52	64.21	42	29.87	___	___
52.5	64.56	42.5	30.05	___	___
53	65.61	43	30.58	___	___
53.5	65.96	43.5	30.76	___	___
54	67.00	44	31.29	___	___
54.5	67.35	44.5	31.47	___	___
55	68.40	45	32.00	___	___
55.5	68.75	45.5	32.18	___	___
56	69.80	46	32.71	___	___
56.5	70.15	46.5	32.89	___	___
57	71.19	47	33.42	___	___
57.5	71.54	47.5	33.60	___	___
58	72.59	48	34.13	___	___
58.5	72.94	48.5	34.31	___	___
59	73.99	49	34.84	___	___
59.5	74.34	49.5	35.02	___	___
60	75.39	50	35.56	___	___

5. Add constants A and B. Then subtract constant C. This will give your percentage of body fat. Plug the constants into the following equation:

A _____ + B _____ – C _____ = your percentage of body fat _____

6. Now take your percentage of body fat and multiply it by your weight. This gives you your fat body mass.

% body fat _____ x weight _____ = fat body mass _____

7. Subtract fat body mass from weight, giving your lean body mass.

Weight _____ – fat body mass _____ = lean body mass _____

8. Multiply your lean body mass by 0.6. This tells you your daily protein requirement in grams.

Lean body mass _____ x 0.6 = grams _____. This is your daily
protein requirement.

Protein Needs

The cornerstone of this meal plan is your daily protein requirement. Each day, your body needs a certain amount of protein for your vital tissues to function properly. Our goal in this plan is to promote lean body mass to reduce insulin resistance, and you can't do that without protein.

Although Americans do tend to eat enough protein overall, many of us fail to pay attention to our daily requirements. You may have figured that if you eat extra protein tomorrow, it's no big deal if you don't get enough today. But for those of us who are prone to insulin resistance—up to 75 percent of us in the United States, according to recent studies from Stanford—eating enough protein every day is critical to maintaining good health and increasing fertility.

Your daily protein requirement, as you've just determined by checking the chart or applying the formula, is the number of grams of protein your body needs each day. You'll add up the grams of protein in your meals and snacks throughout the day to make sure you've achieved this requirement. Protein comes from many sources, such as meat, soy, and eggs. Most animal products are complete proteins, whereas most plant products are incomplete proteins. (Soybeans are the exception: they are complete proteins.)

While it may be harder for vegetarians to increase their protein intake and get all their essential amino acids, this goal is very achievable. We don't encourage you to eat meat if you object to doing so. Nuts and legumes are excellent sources of protein and a variety of other favorable nutrients. Additionally, you can use protein powders as a supplement. You might whip up a fruit smoothie with protein powder in the morning to have a well-balanced meal in one cup. Just remember to check your amino acids; the essential amino acids that are missing in one plant source may be found in another, so you'll have to be vigilant about eating enough variety to get all nine essential amino acids. (You don't need to worry about eating all nine of them at every meal; just don't habitually skip any.)

ESTIMATES OF AMINO-ACID REQUIREMENTS FOR ADULTS [1]

Histidine	10 milligrams per kilogram (10 mg/kg)
Isoleucine	10 mg/kg
Leucine	14 mg/kg
Lysine	12 mg/kg
Methionine plus cystine	13 mg/kg
Phenylalanine plus tyrosine	14 mg/kg
Threonine	7 mg/kg
Tryptophan	3.5 mg/kg
Valine	10 mg/kg

Everything listed in the chart is an essential amino acid, with the exception of cystine and tyrosine, which are nonessential amino acids. The required amounts of the nine essential amino acids must be provided in the diet, but because cystine can replace approximately 30 percent of the requirement for methionine, and tyrosine about 50 percent of the requirement for phenylalanine, those two are included in the measurements.

Be vigilant when you read food labels. Some foods that contain plenty of protein are, unfortunately, not great options, because of the amount of fat that comes tagging along. A cup of whole milk, for example, has eight grams of protein, but almost nine grams of fat (more than half of which is saturated fat). By the way, if you haven't tried skim milk in the past few years, the time has come to give it another shot—it's much improved from the watery, tasteless stuff you may remember from your youth.

You probably needn't worry about getting too much protein. One study did find that a high-protein diet (more than 95 grams per day) over a long period of time can make you more vulnerable to forearm bone fractures—but the same study also found that women who ate the most protein (about 110 grams per day) had a lower risk of heart attack and of death from heart disease.[2] If you have kidney or liver problems, though, a very high-protein diet can aggravate them, so check in with your doctor if this is a concern for you.

PROTEIN SOURCES[3]

Food	Serving Weight (in Grams)	Serving Portion	Protein Content (in Grams)
Halibut	159	½ fillet	42.44
Salmon	155	½ fillet	42.33
Roasted turkey	140	1 cup	41.05
Tuna salad	205	1 cup	32.88
Soybeans (boiled, unsalted)	172	1 cup	28.62
Low-fat cottage cheese (1% milk fat)	226	1 cup	28.00
Couscous (dry)	173	1 cup	22.07
Pinto beans (boiled, unsalted)	171	1 cup	15.41
Chicken vegetable soup	240	1 cup	12.31
Plain yogurt (low-fat)	227	8-oz. container	11.92
Extra-lean ham	56.7	2 slices	9.80

MICE AND MEN

You may have heard a rumor that a diet with more than 20 percent protein can harm fertility. This just isn't true, but let's examine where that rumor came from. In June 2004, a well-respected embryologist presented some of his research to the European Society of Human Reproduction and Embryology. He and his team had conducted a study in which they fed groups of mice diets of 25 percent protein or 14 percent protein for four weeks before mating them. The researchers found that among the mice in the higher-protein group, 65 percent of the embryos developed into fetuses, whereas among the mice in the lower-protein group, 81 percent of the embryos developed into fetuses.[4]

In his presentation, the embryologist said, "It would be prudent to advise couples who are trying to conceive, either naturally or via ART [assisted reproductive therapy], to ensure that the woman's protein intake is less than 20 percent of her total energy consumption."

That's a big leap to take.

First of all, this study was done on mice. Humans are not mice. Our bodies and reproductive systems work differently. (Actually, our reproductive system is most closely related to that of the sheep, so fertility research is often conducted on sheep.) Our digestive systems work differently from mice's, too—mice tend to eat a very low-protein diet of grains rather than going out for surf 'n' turf at Sizzler too often. A high-protein diet is not at all natural for mice.

To be fair, I should add that the presenter did qualify his remarks by stating, "One has to start off with the assumption that the mouse is generally more of a herbivorous animal than we are and, like a cow, is less able to metabolize high amounts of protein." But this got lost in some of the media rush, which led off with headlines like "High-Protein Diet May Ruin Chance of Pregnancy!" That's inaccurate, and not something you need to take seriously.

It also should be noted that this was only one study. Other studies done with humans show improved fertility function when the diet contains somewhat higher protein ratios. Our data show better ovulation with this plan when it is directly compared with a diet following the Food Guide Pyramid, which has relatively lower protein content.

Some programs recommend 50 percent or more protein in the total diet; this would probably become a problem for fertility. When the body has an excess of protein, it secretes more insulin to break down the ketone bodies. That's why we recommend a balanced diet of equal amounts of protein and carbs, which will keep your insulin stabilized.

NOT ENOUGH PROTEIN

Although it's not hard to get enough protein overall in a day, it can be tough to incorporate enough protein into each meal and snack.

READY-MADE PROTEIN PRODUCTS

The easiest trick is to pick up protein bars and shakes. Many of them are formulated with proper ratios of protein to carbohydrates. Just check the nutritional label to make sure the proportions are right, then stock up. Keep them handy, especially in the car, in your purse, or in your briefcase for when you're away from home.

But you need to be careful—not all meal bars are created equal!

An independent research laboratory (Consumerlab.com) tested many brands, comparing the true nutritional content with what their "Nutritional Facts" label stated. The results were mostly good—Consumerlab found that most products lived up to the claims on their labels. However, three products failed. According to the tests, one of the protein bars that was analyzed contained 33 percent more carbohydrate than was listed (an extra 8.3 grams), another low-carb bar contained 50 percent more saturated fat than was listed (an extra gram), and another energy-nutrition bar contained approximately 27 percent more saturated fat (an extra 0.8 gram) than was listed.

Some bars that scored high marks were Met-Rx Sports Nutrition Protein Plus bar, Protein Revolution by Pure Protein, Carb Minders' High Protein Bar for Low-Carb Diets, Carb Solutions High Protein Bar for Low Carb Diets and Good Mornings! Breakfast and Lunch Bars, Power Bar CarbSelects and Performance Energy Bar, and XS Power Nutrition Energy Bars.

HOW TO CHOOSE A PROTEIN POWDER

Then there's protein powder. Most powders have about 10 grams of protein in a scoop. They are of varying quality, and you may have to experiment a bit to find one you like, but they can certainly help you add enough protein to a meal.

First, make sure the powder has an adequate amount of all nine essential amino acids per serving (check the estimated requirements on page 24). Whey protein powders are the most popular and correctly balanced in terms of amino acid distribution. They also have benefits for your immune system. Micellar casein protein powder releases amino acids more slowly and steadily, though.

Next, make sure you can stand the taste and texture! Some protein powders are chalky and thick, while others are smoother and blander, and they come in just about as many flavors as ice cream does. Try to buy a few small samples so that you can decide which one is your favorite. You can mix the powder into just about any drink—plain water, skim milk, juice, or a smoothie. You can also add the powder to oatmeal, yogurt, or pudding.

Some powders are far easier to mix than others, and you can't always trust the advertisements. You may find that the ones touted as "easy to mix" actually clump up and stick to the sides of your blender. Ideally, you want a powder that doesn't require a blender at all; you should be able to mix it to a smooth consistency with a spoon.

Pay attention, too, to the amount of sugar in a protein powder. Most powders are low in sugar, but a few (mainly meant for bodybuilders who are trying to gain weight) are not.

Many protein powders are milk derivatives, but you can find no-lactose and low-lactose products if lactose is a concern for you. Soy proteins are generally the best options in that case.

If you're not used to getting enough protein, you may experience mild gastrointestinal side effects, like bloating and flatulence, at first. If these effects persist, try switching brands; it seems that some protein powders tend to be harder to digest than others.

SWITCH YOUR SNACKS
TO GET MORE PROTEIN

Try to establish new habits regarding snack foods if you're not meeting your protein requirements. Replace potato chips and pretzels with nuts. Keep in mind, though, that cashews and macadamia nuts are very high in fat, so watch your portion size! Peanuts tend to be fairly high in carbs. Almonds are a great choice because they have a roughly equal balance of protein, carbs, and fat.

Beef jerky is good if you're looking for a more substantial snack, and low-fat cottage cheese goes well with many fruits and berries.

Carb Needs

Balancing daily protein intake with an equal amount of carbs, gram for gram, while keeping starchy carbs to a minimum, has been shown to be the lowest stimulus for insulin secretion. So, considering that our aim is to keep your insulin levels low and increase your fertility, we want you to eat the same amount of carbs as you do protein. You'll measure in grams, so all you have to do is eat an equal number of grams of carbs and proteins. It's critical, though, that you do this at every meal and snack. It's this even balance at each meal that causes the lowest insulin secretion, thus keeping insulin from getting in the way of ovulation and implantation. Therefore, don't try to load up on protein during one meal so that you can have extra carbs at a later time. You don't want to negate the hard work you're doing by letting your insulin fly high because you felt like having a pasta-and-potato cake with raspberry syrup!

When it comes to carbs, what matters is quality. You want to choose foods that your body will absorb more slowly, thus keeping the insulin from running amok. The table "Carb Sources" on pages 31–32 lists examples of some favorable and unfavorable carbs.

While there are a few forbidden fruits, most produce is completely acceptable, and you are encouraged to eat it. In addition to having a low glycemic load, most produce is full of other important nutrients. Fresh, frozen, and canned fruits and veggies are all acceptable. Unless you buy organic food, the produce you eat (from a grocery store) is no better than most canned and frozen fruits and vegetables, which retain just as many (if not more) vitamins and minerals. Usually, canned and frozen foods are taken right from the field and processed, preserving greater amounts of vitamin C and other nutrients. Since there's quite a lag from farm to market for most of our fresh produce, these important vitamins and minerals begin to break down.

This doesn't mean we're encouraging you to eat only canned foods—certainly, canned green beans taste different from fresh green beans—but they're all acceptable alternatives. Just be sure to check out the sugar and salt contents of canned goods. Fortunately, there are many no-salt options, and there are products available with reduced sugar or 100 percent juice.

Dried fruits and vegetables are a different story altogether. The process by which produce is commercially dried leeches it of its valuable nutrients. These foods become, essentially, empty calories. However, produce that is dehydrated in your oven or by other home drying methods is completely acceptable. We'll just caution you, from experience, that you might eat a lot more dried fruit than you would fresh, and the carbs add up quickly!

The most restrictive area of this diet is starches, though there are some favorable pastas, rice, and other grains. If there's a specific grain you're interested in researching, check out www.glycemic index.com. This site provides both the glycemic index and the glycemic load for many foods. If the glycemic load is less than 20, it's okay to try. Just remember to keep in check the ratio of grams of protein to grams of carbs.

And don't forget that your drinks count, too! One of my patients, Stephanie, reminded me of this sometimes overlooked factor. Stephanie was 28 years old, five feet one inch, and 115 pounds, with two prior pregnancies when she came to see me unable to achieve a third. Her second pregnancy had had several complications. She developed gestational diabetes, and the fetus was diagnosed with a neural-tube defect. After intrauterine fetal surgery, the child was doing well; however, at two years postpartum, Stephanie had no menstrual cycles.

Upon evaluation, we noted that her ovaries appeared to be polycystic. A screening showed no diabetes but did show marked hypoglycemia two hours after a glucose load, which is consistent with insulin resistance and hyperinsulinemia. What might be causing this? After some questioning, she revealed that she drank six sodas per day (a total of 275 grams of carbohydrates) and that her typical lunch consisted of a soda and a Snickers bar. Mystery solved. She began the diet and exercise regimen we recommended and achieved monthly spontaneous menses in the first two months.

CARB SOURCES

Low Glycemic Index (Favorable)	Grams per Ounce	High Glycemic Index (Less Favorable)	Grams per Ounce
Vegetables		**Vegetables**	
Artichoke	2	Acorn squash	4
Asparagus	1	Baked beans	6
Bean (black)	17	Carrots	8
Bean (green)	2	Corn	6
Bell pepper	2	Lima beans	6
Broccoli	2	Potato	13
Brussels sprouts	3	Refried beans	5
Cabbage	2	Sweet potato	7
Cauliflower	1	**Fruits**	
Celery	1	Banana	7 (28 g/banana)
Cucumber	1	Cranberries	14 g/cup
Collard greens	2	Dates	20
Eggplant	2	Fig	6
Lettuce (iceberg)	1	Mango	5 (35 g/mango)
Lettuce (romaine)	1	Papaya	3 (30 g/papaya)
Mushrooms	1	Prune	20
Onions	3	Raisins	130 g/cup

(continued)

CARB SOURCES (continued)

Low Glycemic Index (Favorable)	Grams per Ounce	High Glycemic Index (Less Favorable)	Grams per Ounce
Peas	2	**Grains**	
Spinach	1	Bagel	40 g/bagel
Tomato	2	Biscuit	25 g/biscuit
Yellow squash	3	Bread, white (slice)	13
Zucchini	1	Breadstick	7 g/stick
Fruits		Bun (hamburger)	35 g/bun
Apple	4 (about 21 g/apple)	Cereal, refined (dry)	25
Apricots	3	Croissant	15
Blueberries	20 g/cup	Crouton	22 g/cup
Cantaloupe	2	Donut	30–60 g/donut
Cherries	19 g/cup	Grits	30 g/cup
Grapefruit	3 (12 g/half)	Muffin	30 g/muffin
Grapes	4 g/10 grapes	Noodles (egg)	40
Kiwi	4 (12 g/kiwi)	Pancake	15 g/pancake
Lemon	2	Pasta, white	20
Lime	3	Popcorn	15
New Potatoes	18	Rice, white	40 g/cup
Orange	3 (15 g/orange)	Tortilla (corn)	10 g/tortilla
Peach	3 (10 g/peach)	Tortilla (flour)	23 g/tortilla
Pineapple	4	Waffle	15 g/waffle
Plum	4 (8 g/plum)	**Sauces**	
Raspberries	14 g/cup	Barbecue	10
Strawberries	10 g/cup	Ketchup	7
Watermelon	6 g/cup	Honey	23
Grains		Jelly	10
Bread, whole-grain (slice)	15	Syrup	26
Buckwheat	20		
Couscous, dry	21		
Oatmeal (slow-cooking)	18 g/cup		
Pasta, protein-enriched	20		
Quinoa, dry	20		
Rice, high-amylose	35 g/cup		
Rice, wild, dry	20		

FREE FOODS

On this plan, there are some vegetables you can eat as much as you want of. They are chock-full of nutrients. After you've balanced your carbs and proteins at each meal, if you're still hungry, these are the "free foods" you're allowed to eat whenever you like (with meals or snacks).

You can eat them fresh, grilled, roasted, sautéed, in a salad—however you like. Experiment with olive oil, vinegar, and spices to dress your veggies, as opposed to coating these goodies in butter. In Mediterranean countries, where olive oil is used abundantly and butter and margarine are used rarely, heart disease is much less a threat than it is in the United States. Although that's certainly not the only reason there are fewer cases of heart disease in the Mediterranean countries, many experts believe it's an important factor. And for fertility purposes, olive oil has an even more compelling benefit: it lowers insulin resistance. There are many terrific olive oils on the market that add a ton of flavor, even when used in small amounts. Brush veggies lightly with olive oil before and during roasting and grilling. Some of the best dressings can be made with just olive oil and vinegar: our basic olive oil vinaigrettes are just two parts olive oil to one part vinegar.

The only restrictions associated with the free foods are on the cream and cheese sauces you may want to use with them. While they can be tasty, these sauces may have hidden carbs and usually contain quite a bit of saturated fat. The vegetables themselves are "free," but the dressings and sauces you use on them are not. Certainly, eat these combinations in moderation if you enjoy them, but you must count the grams of protein, carbs, and fat in anything you add to the vegetables in your diet plan.

Here's the list of freebies:

Artichoke (both leaves and heart)
Asparagus
Beet greens
Bok choy

Broccoli

Brussels sprouts

Cabbage (green and red)

Cauliflower

Celery

Chicory

Chinese cabbage

Chives

Collard greens

Cucumbers

Dandelion greens

Eggplants

Endives

Escarole

Fennel

Garlic

Green beans

Kale

Kohlrabi

Lettuce (avoid iceberg; it has fewer nutrients than other types of
lettuce)

Mushrooms

Mustard greens

Onions

Parsley

Peas

Peppers (all kinds, including chilies)

Radishes

Seaweed

Spinach

Summer squash

Swiss chard

Tomatillos

Tomatoes

Turnip greens

Turnips

Watercress

Yellow squashes (summer, spaghetti, etc.)

Zucchini

CONQUERING CRAVINGS

If you consider yourself a chocoholic, you're in good company. Chocolate is considered the most craved food in the world, with as many as 40 percent of women reporting a craving for it.

For those who simply must have it, chocolate mouth sprays such as Binge Buster (www.bingebuster.com) are available to provide the flavor without adding carbs. Sugar-free hot cocoa and pudding are also excellent choices. Add some protein powder to the mix to balance the carbs from the milk or use a low-carb dairy product.

In general, quitting anything cold turkey doesn't work well, and besides, we don't want you to feel deprived of a favorite food. If you allow yourself a little bit of indulgence, you're likely to have better long-term control. Otherwise, you might just feel so deprived that you go off the deep end and eat a whole pan of brownies at the next family picnic.

Many candy producers now make carb-free chocolates that are a great alternative to their high-carb counterparts. When possible, stick to these. And instead of really falling off the wagon with a slice of double-chocolate explosion cake, why not try a couple of chocolate-covered strawberries and a protein shake?

THE MUNCHIES FOR THE CRUNCHIES

The other common food craving is for chips and crackers: potato chips, Doritos, Fritos—you know, those shiny bags that are right in your face when you pass a vending machine or stand in line at the deli counter. Resist, resist!

If it's the crunch you crave (and it often is, because crunchiness is a tension-releaser), try apple slices or carrot or celery sticks instead.

Soy crisps will also provide that satisfying crunch—along with some rewarding protein.

There are many low-carb chips available; they're not perfect, but at least they're better than typical chips. Be vigilant about those portion sizes, though—it may be smart to divide a bag of chips into several storage bags so that you don't rely on impulsive judgments. When you're engrossed in a movie, it's easy to lose track and eat a whole bag of chips. Even soy crisps have about 17 grams of carbs per serving, so if you eat two or three servings, you haven't done yourself any good by picking the "healthier" version.

Fat Needs

Remember what we said earlier about fat being an essential part of our diets—please don't eliminate something your body needs! While carbs are the culprit emphasized most recently, fat has long been cast as the villain to those trying to lose weight. No-fat and low-fat diets have been a trend for years, but with mostly unimpressive results. Why? Because sooner or later, people realize that they're really hungry! Without fat to turn off the appetite switch, these diets make most people feel terribly deprived.

Compared with carbs, fats have very little effect on insulin; and fats are very energy-rich, though they have about twice as many calories per gram. We're more conservative about fat than some of the currently popular low-carb diets, but we aren't too restrictive, either. We recommend that you consume about half the number of grams of fat per meal or snack compared with the number of grams of proteins or carbs.

Just as with carbs, though, the type of fat is an important consideration. There are three main types of naturally occurring dietary fats: saturated, monounsaturated, and polyunsaturated. Humans have invented a fourth variation: hydrogenated fats. Here's a sampling of which foods fall into which categories.

TYPES OF FATS

Saturated Fats	Monounsaturated Fats	Polyunsaturated Fats	Hydrogenated Fats
Butter	Olive oil	Corn oil	Margarine
Egg yolks	Canola oil	Safflower oil	Shortening
Meat	Peanut oil	Sunflower oil	Deep-frying fats
Whole milk	Avocados	Sunflower seeds	
Coconut oil	Most nuts	Soybeans	
Palm oil	———	Sesame seeds	

Studies indicate that you should limit the saturated and trans monounsaturated fats in your diet. Polyunsaturated fats and those containing omega-3 fatty acids are more favorable choices and are readily found in fish and some vegetables.

FAT SOURCES

High in Monounsaturated Fatty Acids (Good)	Grams	High in Saturated Fatty Acids (Not so Good)	Grams
Almonds	14 g/oz	Mayonnaise	11 g/tsp
Avocado	5 g/oz	Sesame oil	14 g/tsp
Canola oil	14 g/tsp	Walnuts	17 g/oz
Macadamia nuts	20 g/oz	Bacon	4 g/strip
Olive oil	14 g/tsp	Butter	4 g/tsp
Olives	5 g/10 olives	Cream	5 g/oz
Peanut butter	9 g/tsp	Cream cheese	10 g/oz
Peanut oil	14 g/tsp	Lard	26 g/oz
Peanuts	14 g/oz	Vegetable shortening (Crisco)	12 g/tbsp

Your Daily Food Schedule

Now that we've discussed the basic macronutrients and their functions, to put theory into practice, we'll need a specific daily food plan.

Eat More Often

Yes, you read that right. Americans typically eat three big meals over a span of 9 to 10 hours, leaving 14 to 15 hours of fasting until the next day's first meal. Think about it—if you eat dinner at 6 p.m. and then don't eat again until breakfast at 8:30 the next morning, you've fasted for 14½ hours—more than half a day.

Our goal will be to break the "feed-fast" cycle to achieve smoother energy usage and improve your insulin sensitivity. This means that you get to eat more often!

We recommend three main meals and two snacks per day. The first snack can be eaten either late in the morning or in mid-afternoon, depending on your schedule or preference. The second snack should be consumed less than an hour before bed, so that you'll decrease the time your body is in fasting mode to no more than 10 hours.

When you shift to this pattern of eating, your body will become more efficient at metabolizing caloric intake from the diet. (Many of the "miracle weight-loss" drinks that you take before bed are simply amino acids and herbs. These products help combat the storage mode created by our feed-and-fast eating habits.) Regulating your body's insulin levels and getting a constant source of the body's necessary nutrients will help put you on the right track for improved ovulation and fertility.

Your eating pattern should look like one of the following two scenarios, with carbs and proteins balanced at each meal and snack, and approximately half the amount of fat versus carbs or proteins.

> *Scenario 1 (Optimal, eating about every 3 to 4 hours):*
> Breakfast (as soon as you awaken, not a couple of hours later)
> Mid-morning snack
> Lunch
> Dinner
> Bedtime snack

Scenario 2:
Breakfast
Lunch
Mid-afternoon snack
Dinner
Bedtime snack

You should feel quite satisfied if you're eating five times a day and getting the proper amount of fat in your diet. If not, continue to adjust your food choices and eating patterns to fit your needs. Keep in mind that you should not go longer than eight hours without food on a regular basis.

Thank You, FDA

Now that you know what proportion of grams of protein, carbs, and fats to eat at each meal and snack, how are you going to figure out how many grams of each are in your food? Thanks to the Food and Drug Administration (FDA), all you have to do is read the labels.

As you're probably aware, the FDA requires many food packages to have a label called "Nutritional Facts" that lists the number of grams of fat, protein, and carbs in each item. For our purposes, the grams of protein and fat can be read as listed. To figure out the amount of carbs that will count toward your carb requirement, however, requires just a tiny bit of math. Take the number of grams of carbs listed, then subtract the number of grams of fiber. Simple carbs with a high GI are listed as "sugars" and should be limited.

Even a soda bottle has "Nutrition Facts" on its label. Read the label and try not to weep.

Now for a gentle reminder. Please note that the grams on the label are listed "per serving." Even though a package may look like one serving to most of us, it may quite possibly be two or three servings according to the manufacturer. (What? The manufacturer thinks two cookies are a serving? Yes, they're cruel that way.) It does you no good to calculate your nutritional values and then eat double the amount you allotted. If you're going to eat two or three servings of a particular food, you need to account for that when you're checking your nutrient proportions.

Here's an example of a label, to give you an idea of what to look for and how to figure the amount of carbs that count toward raising your blood sugar:

Nutrition Facts

Serving Size 1/2 cup (114g)
Servings Per Container 4

Amount Per Serving

Calories 90   Calories from Fat 30

	% Daily Value*
Total Fat 3g	**5%**
Saturated Fat 0g	**0%**
Cholesterol 0mg	**0%**
Sodium 300mg	**13%**
Total Carbohydrate 13g	**4%**
Dietary Fiber 3g	**12%**
Sugars 3g	
Protein 3g	

Vitamin A 80% • Vitamin C 60%

Calcium 4% • Iron 4%

* Percent Daily Values are based on a 2,000 calorie diet. Your daily values may be higher or lower depending on your calorie needs:

	Calories:	2,000	2,500
Total Fat	Less than	65g	80g
Sat Fat	Less than	20g	25g
Cholesterol	Less than	300mg	300mg
Sodium	Less than	2,400mg	2,400mg
Total Carbohydate		300g	375g
Dietary Fiber		25g	30g

Calories per gram:
Fat 9 • Carbohydrate 4 • Protein 4

You get to subtract the fiber from the carb count, because fiber is good for your digestive processes and does not contribute to raising your blood sugar. Yippee—free carbs!

For protein and fat measurements, simply take the grams listed and multiply by the number of servings you are going to eat. For carbs, take the grams listed for "Total Carbohydrate," then subtract the grams listed as "Dietary Fiber." Then you take this total and multiply it by your serving size.

We'll look at two different scenarios using the sample label. First, let's say you're going to have the manufacturer's recommended serving size of this item. You'd figure out your nutrient grams as follows:

> **Protein:** 3 g x 1 (serving) = 3 g
>
> **Fat:** 3 g x 1 (serving) = 3 g
>
> **Carbs:** 13 g (total carbs) – 3 g (dietary fiber) = 10 g

Then

> 10 g x 1 (serving) = 10 g

Now let's say you want to have three times the manufacturer's serving size. Then the number of grams you will be ingesting would be calculated like this:

> **Protein:** 3 g x 3 (servings) = 9 g
>
> **Fat:** 3 g x 3 (servings) = 9 g
>
> **Carbs:** 13 g (total carbs) – 3 g (dietary fiber) = 10 g

Then

> 10 g x 3 (servings) = 30 g

Eating Out

When you eat out, you lose some control over what is available, how food is prepared, and how much is served. Even if there are "healthy" choices, it's often hard to select them, because the other choices sound so much better! To stay in charge of the situation and avoid overindulging, keep these tips in mind:

1. **Choose restaurants that offer healthy fare.** Avoid all-you-can-eat buffets. Look at the menu before sitting down, and check to see if there's a "low-carb" section. More and more restaurants now offer several low-carb options.

2. **Avoid arriving ravenously hungry.** If you're at a holiday party, everything will look good, and food will probably be everywhere you look. If you haven't eaten in hours, you're likely to overload your plate or keep going back for more. If you're at a restaurant, you will be likely to overindulge in appetizers and bread while you wait for your meal to come. If you do order an appetizer, a salad is a good choice (many appetizers are either heavily breaded or prepared in heavy sauces; look for choices that are not prepared this way). To avoid falling prey to this situation, have a light snack before you go—a piece of fruit, a small container of yogurt, a handful of nuts, or a string cheese. The same applies to shopping for groceries, by the way—Don't shop while hungry! You're much more likely to fill your cart with anything that makes your mouth water.

3. **Decide what you really want, then balance your choices.** There's no need to forbid yourself to eat your favorite foods at your favorite restaurants. This is especially true if eating out is a rare treat for you. Besides, if you don't let yourself eat what you really want, you'll leave feeling deprived and unsatisfied, and you may overeat later. If you have your heart set on a rich dessert that's loaded with carbohydrates and fat, balance it out by ordering an entrée of lean protein and vegetables (like a grilled chicken salad with light dressing or a piece of grilled fish with steamed vegetables). If you really want that high-fat burger, skip the greasy fries and enjoy some carrot sticks or fresh fruit with it instead. Balance is the key!

4. **Saladify it.** Don't be afraid to ask for substitutions; if a meal comes with fries, potatoes, or rice, ask if you can order a better alternative. And most entrées can be turned into dinner salads—instead of having meat on top of a bed of rice or pasta, ask to have it tossed into a salad. If you're normally not a "salad person," you may

be surprised to find that salads really can fill you up. As an extra bonus, the roughage helps your digestive tract work more smoothly.

5. **Watch those portions.** If your willpower isn't feeling strong, you can ask the waiter or waitress to bring you a smaller portion. Ask for one scoop of rice instead of two, or a small order of fries instead of the medium or large order that usually comes with the meal. Otherwise, you can ask for two plates. As soon as your meal arrives, split it into two plates: the one you're going to eat now and the one you'll either throw away, give to someone else, or bring home as leftovers. Put that second plate far away from you, give it away, or ask for it to be wrapped immediately so it's not in your face and tempting you.

6. **Take your time.** Slow down, put your fork down between bites, and chew well.

7. **Drink water.** And lots of it! Drink a tall glass of water before you start eating and several glasses during your meal. It'll help you feel full.

8. **Signal "The End."** Take deliberate steps to end your meal. Get up and brush your teeth, suck on a sugar-free mint, chew sugarless gum, or drink a tall glass of water to cue yourself that the meal is over. Get any remaining food out of your sight, so even if your friends aren't finished yet or want to stick around at the table to chat, you won't be tempted to keep eating.

What About Meals on the Go?

Fast-food restaurants are required to make nutritional facts available to customers. Just ask the people taking your order for their restaurants' nutritional profile. The FDA is working on requiring other restaurants to provide the same information.

Surprisingly, many restaurants (especially chains) and food counters already do have this information available if you request it, even though it's not required yet. Handy little books with the nutritional contents of meats, fruits, vegetables, and more are also available at most bookstores and grocery stores.

Go Organic

We encourage you to choose organic products when they are available and your budget permits. Important research shows that organic foods contain higher nutrients than nonorganic foods. Additionally, mitochondria, critical structures for combating insulin resistance and improving metabolism, are highly susceptible to the influences of paraquat, paration, donoseb, and 2-4-D, chemicals commonly used in conventional farming. As of October 2002, the U.S. Department of Agriculture (USDA) enacted national standards for foods grown in the United States and overseas: Farmers must meet these standards if their food is to be labeled organic.

According to the National Organic Program of the USDA:

> Organic food is produced by farmers who emphasize the use of renewable resources and the conservation of soil and water to enhance environmental quality for future generations. Organic meat, poultry, eggs, and dairy products come from animals that are given no antibiotics or growth hormones. Organic food is produced without using most conventional pesticides; fertilizers made with synthetic ingredients or sewage sludge; bioengineering; or ionizing radiation. Before a product can be labeled "organic," a government-approved certifier inspects the farm where the food is grown to make sure the farmer is following all the rules necessary to meet USDA organic standards. Companies that handle or process organic food before it gets to your local supermarket or restaurant must be certified, too.

If you see a circular label that says "USDA Organic," the food has been certified as at least 95 percent organic. There's a higher tier, too: foods may be labeled "100 percent organic." If only some ingredients in a food are organic, that can be stated on the package (e.g., "made with organic strawberries and blueberries"). It's illegal for foods from uncertified producers to have the word "organic" on the package.

Although there used to be a large difference in price between organic and conventional produce, the gap is narrowing, and you may be pleased to find that as demand has increased, many organic foods are now more affordable. Organic foods are readily available at most grocery stores and health food stores.

H_2O—Way to Go

Don't forget to drink your water: eight 8-oz. glasses per day at minimum. Very few of us drink enough water each day. Before you eat, be sure to drink a glass of water. This will help you feel less hungry. Some nutritionists speculate that one of the reasons people overeat is that they are actually thirsty, not hungry. They mistake their bodies' cues of thirst for cues of hunger. They keep eating because they haven't squelched the hunger pains and their bodies aren't satisfied. But the problem is that they weren't hungry in the first place—they mistook their bodies' cues and were eating when they should have been drinking.

We recommend that you drink filtered tap water. Unfortunately, we don't have an opportunity to do an individual water analysis on every water system. Many city water systems produce excellent tap water that doesn't need to be filtered. If you have the time and energy, investigate the quality of the water from your local system. Most water companies readily provide this information.

If you prefer bottled water, go ahead and drink it; just be aware that the jury is still out on the long-term interaction of water with plastic bottles. If you can tolerate the taste, stick to filtered tap water. If you know you are going to be away from home for a while and will be unsure of the available water sources, carry a water bottle with you. If you are traveling or just busy and all that is available is bottled water, you might opt for water bottled in glass. If water in a plastic bottle is all that is available, certainly pick that over soda or juice.

Vitamins with Verve—and Minerals

In addition to your meals, you'll also want to take one well-rounded multivitamin, preferably from an organic source.

Folate

Make sure that the multivitamin contains at least 400 micrograms (mcg.) of folate or folic acid. If you're even thinking of becoming pregnant, you should begin watching your folate levels closely, making sure you're getting enough every day. Folate is a key nutrient during pregnancy; cases of neural-tube defects are reduced by 50 to 70 percent when women get enough folic acid. The most important time to prevent these defects is during the first few weeks after conception.

You can take folate as part of a prenatal vitamin or as a separate supplement. Women who've already had children with neural-tube defects or have an increased risk for such fetal defects should take at least 4,000 mcg. per day.

If you don't get folate in your vitamin, make sure it's in your diet. One bowl of fortified cereal may be enough to meet the daily requirement; other good sources include lentils, spinach, orange juice, and brussels sprouts.

Iron

Pregnant women are advised to take 30 mg. of iron per day in the second and third trimesters to prevent iron-deficiency anemia. This

can be part of a multivitamin and can be taken at bedtime or between meals with juice or water. For anemic women, your doctor
can tell you the appropriate therapeutic dose: usually 60–120 mg.
per day.

Calcium

You'll need at least 1,500 mg. of calcium per day to maintain your
bone density and to prepare for milk production. The baby will take
all it needs for its bone growth, so the extra calcium is really needed
to protect Mom. You don't want the baby to leech all the calcium out
of your body!

You can get your calcium in supplements, in prenatal vitamins, or
from your diet. Low-fat dairy products (milk, yogurt, and cheese) are
good dietary sources, and orange juice is often fortified with calcium.

Many calcium supplements are available, but taking three Extra-
Strength TUMS will give you all the calcium you need, and it also
helps relieve reflux heartburn.

Vitamins C and E

Your body will have an increased need for vitamin C during pregnancy. At least 75 mg. per day is what the Food and Nutrition Board
of the Institute of Medicine recommends for nonpregnant adult
women. Pregnant women are advised to get at least 85 mg. daily.
These requirements were raised in 2000.[5]

Sufficient amounts of vitamin C and vitamin E may be associated
with reducing several risks during pregnancy including preeclampsia, gestational diabetes, and premature rupture of membranes.

Good dietary sources of vitamin C include citrus fruits, berries,
asparagus, broccoli, cauliflower, kale, and fortified cereals. To retain
the most vitamin C, eat your fruits and vegetables raw.

Prenatal Vitamins

Most prenatal vitamins will contain the above items as well as a full spectrum of B vitamins and antioxidants. Even if you're just thinking about becoming pregnant, it's a good idea to ask your doctor to prescribe a prenatal vitamin for you.

One common side effect of prenatal vitamins is stomach upset. If this affects you, you can switch to a different prenatal vitamin or to a general multivitamin. Children's vitamins are often very well tolerated and effective in adults.

Just be wary of the quality of the vitamins you are using. Vitamins are *not* all the same, and the FDA does not test dietary supplements to be sure they meet the claims on their labels or to check that they're free of impurities. Luckily, an independent research laboratory (Consumerlab.com) tested 47 brands of multivitamins, including several prenatal and women's vitamins, and published the results.

Eleven of the 47 failed the tests for accuracy of doses, reproducibility, or absorption.

Those achieving high scores included Rainbow Light's Just Once Naturals, Prenatal One and Women's One Multivitamins, and Nature Made's Essential Woman Complete Multivitamin/Mineral Supplement.

You'll need a paid subscription to view all the results, but you can check out a sampling of the vitamins this laboratory approved at http://www.consumerlab.com/results/multivit.asp.

What to Avoid

Last Call for Alcohol

With regard to alcohol, the debate continues about its effect on insulin resistance. Some studies have concluded that light consumption of alcohol actually helped insulin sensitivity, whereas heavy consumption hindered insulin sensitivity; other studies concluded that alcohol consumption uniformly hinders insulin sensitivity.

But because your goal is to get pregnant, we're recommending the guidelines of the American College of Obstetricians and Gynecologists (ACOG). ACOG advises pregnant women to abstain from alcoholic beverages. Because it could take several weeks for you to find out that you're pregnant, you should play it safe and as soon as you start trying to conceive, treat your body as if you were already pregnant.

Go Unleaded

This just in: it appears caffeine is losing the insulin debate.

For years, researchers have been trying to figure out why coffee seems to actually help insulin sensitivity. Studies have found that people who drink a lot of coffee are at lower risk for type 2 diabetes, for example.[6] For some time, it seemed that caffeine might actually be good for blood sugar.

But that's not true.

Several new studies have found that it's not the caffeine that helps; it's something else in coffee, which is also present in decaffeinated coffee. The caffeine hurts insulin sensitivity. A study done in Canada in 2005 found that ingesting caffeine harmed the insulin sensitivity of lean, obese, and diabetic individuals alike.[7] The results of this study were replicated many times by other researchers.

Now that scientists are aware that caffeine contributes to insulin resistance, they have begun to hypothesize about what it is in coffee that's helpful, and the leading theory right now is that the chlorogenic acids in coffee keep blood sugar levels from spiking. An as yet unpublished study completed at the University of Guelph in Ontario found that decaffeinated coffee drove blood sugar concentrations down in both diabetic and nondiabetic volunteers, whereas regular coffee disrupted blood sugar levels for several hours.[8]

Further, researchers in North Carolina interviewed 104 healthy women who had been trying for three months to get pregnant, and found that women who said they consumed more than the equivalent of one cup of coffee per day were half as likely to become pregnant, per cycle, as women who drank less.[9]

On the basis of past research, ACOG recommends no more than two cups of coffee per day for pregnant women. On the basis of this new research, we recommend that you immediately switch to decaf! Not only will it not hurt; it actually improves your insulin sensitivity. If you find the thought of losing that morning rush horrifying, try mixing half-decaf with half-regular.

Also remember that coffee isn't the only source of caffeine—it's just the only one that has a small "get out of jail free" card because of the substance in coffee that lessens caffeine's negative effects on blood sugar. The other main sources of caffeine are tea, cola drinks, chocolate, hot cocoa, energy drinks, and medications (both prescription and over-the-counter). Even decaf coffee is allowed to have a small amount of caffeine in it. To check your caffeine consumption, use this chart.

COMMON SOURCES OF CAFFEINE[10]

Item	Milligrams of Caffeine	
	Typical	Range*
Coffee (1 cup, 8 fluid ounces)		
Brewed, drip method	85	65–120
Brewed, percolator	75	60–85
Decaffeinated, brewed	3	2–4
Espresso (1 serving, 1 fl. oz.)	40	30–50
Teas (1 cup, 8 fl. oz.)		
Brewed	40	20–90
Instant	28	24–31
Iced (1 glass, 8 fl. oz.)	25	9–50

* For coffee and tea products, the range varies, owing to brewing method, plant variety, brand of product, etc.

Some soft drinks (8 fl. oz.)	24	20–40
"Energy drinks"	80	0–80
Cocoa beverage (8 fl. oz.)	6	3–32
Chocolate milk beverage (8 fl. oz.)	5	2–7
Milk chocolate (1 oz.)	6	1–15
Dark chocolate, semisweet (1 oz.)	20	5–35
Baker's chocolate (1 oz.)	26	26
Chocolate-flavored syrup (1 fl. oz.)	4	4

Caffeine can also interfere with iron absorption, so don't drink coffee or regular tea with your vitamins or supplements. If you want to try to eliminate caffeine from your diet entirely, we won't complain. But if you find that too restrictive, just do your best to keep caffeine levels low, so your blood sugar levels won't look as if they've been jumping on a trampoline all day.

If you're a caffeine addict, be aware that you may go through some mild withdrawal symptoms (headaches, restlessness) for a week or two if you try to quit cold turkey. It's better to wean yourself off caffeine over the course of a week or so.

Your Meal Mission

Your typical meal should consist of a reasonable-size portion of your entrée (usually a source of protein, such as a chicken breast, piece of steak, piece of fish, or single helping of a more elaborately prepared dish) with a side dish of a vegetable, fruit, or salad and a glass of cool, clear water. Snacks should have about a third of the gram content a main meal has and usually should be something lighter, such as cottage cheese with fruit, smoothies, mixed nuts, cold cuts with veggie sticks, or some form of nutrition bar or drink.

Your first meal should take place as soon as possible after you open your eyes in the morning, and your bedtime snack should occur as close to sleep as you can manage. Try to eat every three to four hours, and remember the proportions: approximately equal grams of proteins and carbs during each meal and snack, and half the grams of fat.

This isn't just a "sometimes" plan. For it to have a real impact on your fertility, you need to be diligent about following this program and resetting your body's response to insulin. That doesn't happen overnight, but it can change over a relatively short time. Most people will gain metabolic benefits within the first one to two months of starting the program. Before you get started, however, here is an important point regarding what to expect.

This is not intended to be a rapid weight-loss program. Many people will not lose weight right away when they start this program (and you may not need to lose weight at all). What you will see, however, is your body trimming down. The program is designed to improve your fertility and insulin sensitivity by promoting lean body mass and muscle. Muscle tissue weighs more than fat tissue, so as your body changes, you may notice changes in your physique that do not coincide with a change on the bathroom scale.

Joan was a perfect example of this phenomenon. She returned for a follow-up visit after being on the program for two months. Despite diligently applying these lifestyle changes, she returned very frustrated and felt as though nothing was happening. She stepped on the scale day in and day out and was exactly the same weight as when she started.

I asked whether her clothes fit any better, and she responded emphatically, "Yes! That's just the thing—my waistband is looser and everyone keeps saying I look as if I've lost a ton of weight. But then I have to tell them that I haven't lost a pound!"

Further questioning revealed that her facial hair had lessened, and that her menses were more regular as well. After I strongly reassured her that, by all indications, her metabolic state was improved, and explained that it's normal not to lose weight right away (if at all), her whole outlook changed for the better.

So take heart in devoting yourself to making these lifestyle changes. Your patience and discipline may have the best reward imaginable: a successful pregnancy and a healthy baby.

Three

Sample
Seven-Day Meal Plan
and Recipes

O N THE FOLLOWING pages, you'll find seven suggestions each for breakfasts, lunches, and dinners. I have divided them along the lines of traditional meals, but you can actually use any of the suggestions for any meal—one of our best family meals is pancakes for dinner. So choose whatever suits your palate.

These meals also give you a good idea of how to design your own meals. Each meal doesn't have to be an absolutely perfect balance between protein and carbohydrates. The sample meals are all great examples of ratios that work. Some meals tip slightly toward protein; others tip slightly toward carbs. You probably wouldn't want to overindulge in the meals that are heavy on the fats each and every day, but they are okay sometimes. The idea is to keep each meal in a range where you are taking approximately equal portions of carbohydrates and proteins with each meal, and half that amount of fat.

Sample Breakfasts

Approximate nutritional content is provided in terms of protein, net carbs, and fat for the serving size. Actual counts may vary, depending on some of your selections.

1. **Breakfast on the Go.** Here's one for those days when you have 15 minutes to get dressed, showered, and out of the house. We list this one first because somehow it winds up describing most of our days. This meal-in-a-cup has all the nutrients you need for a fertility-fueled morning.

   - Smoothie with Protein Powder: 1½ cups.
     Nutritional content for strawberry smoothie:
     27 grams protein
     24 grams net carbs (7 grams fiber)
     8 grams total fat

2. **Eggs on the Go-Go.** If you like eggs but don't have time to sit and eat them, here's another one-handed dish for the annals of go-go.

   - Balanced Breakfast Burrito (or "Eggs in a Blanket")
     42 grams protein
     6 grams net carbs (0.1 grams fiber)
     37 grams total fat

3. **Cold Morning—Hot Cereal.** Here's another quick dish that really fills the bill for those days you are craving cereal. I wouldn't take this one on the road, though!

   - Dr. G's protein-rich oatmeal (oatmeal with a scoop of protein powder added)
   - ½ grapefruit
     29 grams protein
     45 grams net carbs (6 grams fiber)
     4 grams total fat

4. **B&E Breakfast.** Eggs and beans are breakfast staples in many cultures. Here's our favorite combo, but be brave—try several combinations and discover the combo that pleases your palate.

   - Huevos Rancheros
   - ½ cup black beans
   - ½ cup cantaloupe
     27 grams protein
     35 grams net carbs (8 grams fiber)
     22 grams total fat

5. **Berry Quick.** Couldn't be simpler.

   - 1 cup low-fat cottage cheese
   - ½ to 1 cup strawberries
     29 grams protein
     18 grams net carbs (4 grams fiber)
     5 grams total fat

6. **Punch up Your Pancakes.** Pancakes with protein? You bet. These fluffy flapjacks have a nutty flavor that will knock your socks off. I wouldn't be surprised if IHOP starts adding this to its menu soon!

   - Power-Packed Pancakes
   - No-sugar-added fruit spread
   - Bacon or sausage. (If you can skip these sides, you'll be healthier for it. It'll mean far less saturated fat. But for some of us, bacon just has to be a part of the program, and it won't affect your fertility on a once-a-week basis.)
     21 grams protein
     23 grams net carbs (3 grams fiber)
     12 grams total fat

7. **Casual Company Breakfast.** Having a few friends over for a morning visit? This quick recipe is sure to please. Even if you're alone, this dish is simple and satisfying.

- Spinach frittata
- ½ cup pineapple
  22 grams protein
  32 grams net carbs (5 grams fiber)
  8 grams total fat

Sample Lunches

Lunch seems to be the easiest meal for people to manage. In our household, lunch seems to revolve around soup, salad, and sandwiches, so here are our suggestions for balanced carbs and proteins. In the recipe section, which follows this section of sample meal plans, you'll also find variations listed underneath the basic recipes.

Here we have seven lunch suggestions. You can have one each day for a week or eat the same one again and again, or choose something from the breakfast or dinner section for lunch instead. Do whatever makes you happy.

1. **Simply Salad.** Most green salads with about 4 oz. of grilled chicken will provide you with a well-balanced meal. Grilled steak, hamburger, and tuna are also terrific on a bed of greens. Have the dressing on the side so you can control how much fat you take in. Choose dressings based on olive oil when you have the chance.

   - Mixed greens with a Dijon vinaigrette with grilled chicken
     35 grams protein
     6 grams net carbs (3 grams fiber)
     14 grams total fat

2. **It's a Wrap.** How can I wrap thee? Let me count the ways. Whatever your favorite sandwich filling, there is a good chance it can be adapted for a lettuce or whole-wheat wrap. Our suggestion is for the conventional at heart, but the more adventurous can create some really great versions. Just make sure you pile on the veggies!

- Ham and cheese wrap
- ¾ cup melon medley
  20 grams protein
  16 grams net carbs (1.2 grams fiber)
  11 grams total fat

3. **Soup's On!** Soups, chilies, and stews can make great balanced lunches. Be careful of soups based on cheese or cream. They can contain hidden carbs and lots of saturated fats. If your bowl doesn't contain a lot of vegetables, you may want to round out your meal with a nice garden salad.

- Four-bean chili
- Side salad
  30 grams protein
  43 grams net carbs (6 grams fiber)
  14 grams total fat

Sample Dinners

1. **Grill It.** Whether you have a George Foreman grill on your counter, a hibachi on your patio, or a Viking on your deck, grilling is great for both your meats and your vegetables regardless of the time of year. You can marinate your food or serve it with just the lightest of seasonings.

- Grilled pork tenderloin
- Grilled vegetables
- ½ cup fruit salad
  44 grams protein
  29 grams net carbs (4 grams fiber)
  12 grams total fat
  (Nutritional content for full recipe)

2. **Forget the Breading—Let's Go Nuts.** Did you grow up in the South, where comfort food is breaded or dipped in batter? Our suggestion is chicken and almonds, but just about any meat with most nuts will work. If you haven't tried this approach to beating the craving for batter, it's worth a try. We now prefer our nutty crust substitute to breading and batter. As an added bonus, with this recipe you don't need to use nearly as much oil.

   • Almond-crusted chicken
   • Orange salsa
   • Fresh steamed snow peas
     41 grams protein
     27 grams net carbs (5 grams fiber)
     13 grams total fat
     (Nutritional content for full recipe)

3. **Stir It Up.** Just about any combo of meat or tofu and veggies, stir-fried, is a great one-dish meal for your fertility diet plan. If you are eating out, be sure to ask if the restaurant uses something to sweeten its sauces. Besides sugar, other sweeteners for stir-fries are honey, molasses, plum sauce, and hoisin. Ask your server if the chef can prepare a stir-fry without the sweetener. If not, ask for other dishes that don't have as much sugar. Cornstarch is another ingredient you need to watch for in restaurant-prepared stir-fries (it packs a whopping 30 grams of carbs per ounce).

   Here's our suggestion for a quick homemade stir-fry. See the recipe for other variations. Remember to skip the rice, or just have a small serving (¼ cup) of brown rice if it's available.

   • Polynesian chicken stir-fry
   • ½ cup couscous
     112 grams protein
     104 grams net carbs (14 grams fiber)
     18 grams total fat
     (Nutritional content for full recipe)

4. **It's Not a Crock!** Crock-pot dinners are great for helping you stay on target. For many people, the motivation for staying on target is strongest in the morning. We wake up and decide that we are going to meet our goals today! But as the day goes on, we face challenges and may struggle to maintain our willpower. A crock-pot dinner is great for helping you to stay on target because you make it when you are motivated, and you don't have to think about what to eat after a long day at the office. It's already there and done! All you have to do is make a fresh tossed salad, and dinner is ready to go without having engaged your brain or your willpower.

   - Swiss steak
   - Steamed green beans
   - Garden tossed salad with vinaigrette
     50 grams protein
     28 grams net carbs (6 grams fiber)
     55 grams total fat
     (Nutritional content for full recipe)

5. **Pleasing Potpie.** I know what you're thinking: "You're kidding, right? A pie?" Well, we wouldn't recommend this one for every night of the week—not because of the carbs, but because making the crust can be rather labor-intensive. Maybe Pillsbury will come out with a low-carb version of piecrust soon. Until then, we have this tasty though time-consuming recipe. When comfort food is a must, and that means potpie to you, this recipe can't be beaten. We have several variations and are sure you can come up with your own version using this basic recipe. This nutty vegan pie crust is so tasty and has such a low glycemic index that you can even squeeze in a small piece of apple pie with a protein shake as one of your snacks.

   - Chicken potpie
   - Caesar salad
     43 grams protein
     58 grams net carbs (13 grams fiber)

78 grams total fat
(Nutritional content for full recipe)

6. **Mouth-Watering Meat Loaf.** Meat loaf doesn't have to be loath-
some. Whether you like patties, balls, or loaves, there are some
great ways to serve ground meats, and most of these recipes can be
adapted to fit your preferred form. You can adapt most of your favorite recipes by substituting almond meal (ground almonds) and
Italian seasoning for the usual bread crumbs. We would recommend staying away from the meatball recipes in which the sauce is
half ketchup and half grape jelly, but most other recipes are great
when you cut back on the sugar or use Splenda as a substitute.
Some of the recipes require such a small amount of sugar per serving that you can prepare them as they are written. We're including
a fun recipe that can be served in meatball form as an interesting
tapa or in meat loaf form for a great little meal.

- Saffron-almond meat loaf
- Spinach salad
- ½ cup cantaloupe
   49 grams protein
   21 grams net carbs (5 grams fiber)
   57 grams total fat
   (Nutritional content for full recipe)

7. **That's a Wrap.** We've wrapped it for breakfast and lunch; we
certainly have to wrap it for dinner. Afraid you'll miss your favorite
fajitas? Whether you crave seafood, chicken, pork, or beef, fear no
more. With all the great low-carb whole-wheat tortillas on the market, you are sure to find something that will work for you. Lettuce is
also a terrific alternative to the traditional high-carb flour and corn
tortillas. When you change the wrap, fajitas are a fast, terrific fertility
food.

- Your favorite fajitas (choose from pork, shrimp, steak, or chicken) with all the fixings (lettuce, cheese, avocado, sour cream)
- ½ cup quinoa
  36 grams protein
  60 grams net carbs (9 grams fiber)
  47 grams total fat
  (Nutritional content for full recipe)

Sample Snacks

Pick two snacks per day: one between meals, the other just before bed.

Part of the key to controlling your insulin is eating every three to four hours, whether you need a mid-morning pick-me-up to make it to lunch, a mid-afternoon snack to make it to dinner, or something to hold you over during your night's rest. Here are some suggestions for quick snacks with balanced carbs and protein.

1. Low-fat mozzarella cheese
   4 or 5 whole-grain crackers
   Red pepper strips or another free veggie
      11 grams protein
      13 grams net carbs (1 gram fiber)
      7 grams total fat

2. ½ apple with peanut butter or almond butter
      9 grams protein
      27 grams net carbs (9 grams fiber)
      16 grams total fat

3. Snack-size container of low-fat cottage cheese
   2 slices of apple or your fill of tomato
      14 grams protein

14 grams net carbs (2 grams fiber)

2 grams total fat

4. 1 cup melon or 1 cup strawberries

    8-oz. protein drink

    11 grams protein

    11 grams net carbs (5 grams fiber)

    1 grams total fat

5. ½ cup LeCarb Ice Cream (Your choice of flavor, but lemon and straw-berry aren't quite as good with almonds!)

    ⅛ cup chopped or slivered almonds

    (Only once per day, and a maximum of two times per week.)

    7 grams protein

    23 grams net carbs (9 grams fiber)

    7 grams total fat

6. Mini-wraps: small ham-and-cheese wrap or another favorite wrap. Just be sure to check your protein intake.

    12 grams protein

    2 grams net carbs (0 grams fiber)

    6 grams total fat

7. Small slice apple pie (vegan crust, low-sugar filling; see recipes)

    8-oz. protein shake

    (You'll be over your carb proportion, but this combo has a very low glycemic index.)

    19 grams protein

    53 grams net carbs (8 grams fiber)

    27 grams total fat

8. Balanced protein-carb bar. Sometimes half of the bar will do the trick.

    20 grams protein

    20 grams net carbs (1 grams fiber)

    9 grams total fat

9. For a special treat, try this:

3 chocolate-dipped strawberries (dark chocolate)

1 cup protein shake

11 grams protein

13 grams net carbs (1 grams fiber)

7 grams total fat

Smoothie

Serves 1 or 2

1 cup frozen strawberries, blueberries, or blackberries

1 8-oz. carton plain Greek yogurt, 2 percent milk fat

1 teaspoon flaxseed oil (optional)

Scoop of protein powder (vanilla or plain)
equivalent to 10 grams protein

2 packets alternative sweetener (to taste)

¼ teaspoon vanilla extract

¼ teaspoon cinnamon (optional)

1 cup ice cubes

PLACE all ingredients in a blender or food processor and process until smooth. If you prefer a thinner consistency, just add a bit of very cold water. If you make the smoothie in a food processor, leave out the ice cubes and add very cold water instead.

27 grams protein

22 grams net carbs (3 grams fiber)

9 grams total fat

Variation

Vegan Smoothie: Substitute (12.3-oz.) box soft tofu, drained, and 2 teaspoons lemon juice for the Greek yogurt.

Breakfast Burrito
Serves 1

Light cooking-oil spray

1 cup cubed ham

3 eggs, beaten

¼ cup shredded cheese
(your choice: cheddar, mozzarella, Swiss, etc.)

Dash of chili powder

Salsa to taste

Large leaf of lettuce

SPRAY skillet with light cooking oil. Heat the skillet and brown the ham. Add the eggs and scramble. Add the shredded cheese and stir in. Add chili powder. Remove from heat.

ADD salsa to taste. Wrap all this in a large lettuce leaf.

42 grams protein

6 grams net carbs (0 grams fiber)

37 grams total fat

Variations

Avocado Burrito: Add chopped avocado with the salsa.

Black Bean Burrito: In lieu of ham, or in addition to the ham if you want, add ½ cup canned, drained black beans. Heat beans in skillet before adding eggs.

Tomatoes and Onions: Add 2 canned tomatoes, chopped, and ¼ cup chopped sautéed onion. Then add ham and proceed as directed in recipe.

43 grams protein

10 grams net carbs (2 grams fiber)

37 grams total fat

Dr. G's Oatmeal

Serves 2

2 cups water

1 cup old-fashioned oats

¼ cup dried apples

*4 scoops vanilla-flavored protein powder
(or the equivalent of 42 grams protein)*

½ teaspoon cinnamon

BRING water to a boil in medium-size saucepan. Add oats and apples, then reduce heat to medium. Cook, stirring occasionally, for five minutes.

REMOVE from heat and add protein powder and cinnamon. Serve with reduced-carb milk. Add more cinnamon to suit your taste.

28 grams protein

33 grams net carbs (5 grams fiber)

4 grams total fat

Huevos Rancheros
Serves 2

2 teaspoons olive oil

2 green onions, chopped

1 fresh tomato, peeled and chopped (or 2 from a can, if good fresh tomatoes are not available)

1 teaspoon fresh oregano (or ¼ teaspoon dried oregano)

1 (4 oz.) can chopped green chilies (or jalapeños)

*6 eggs (We like our eggs over easy,
but this recipe is great with scrambled eggs, too!)*

Dash of salt

Dash of pepper

2 teaspoons chopped fresh cilantro leaves

HEAT oil in a large cast-iron frying pan on medium-high heat. Add the onions and brown for a minute or two. Add the chopped tomato and let cook for a few minutes on medium-high heat until the tomatoes are somewhat cooked and mushy and some of the moisture has evaporated. It's okay if the tomatoes brown a bit. Add the oregano. Add the chili peppers.

CRACK eggs directly into the pan in which the sauce is cooking. Add salt and pepper.

IF you want your eggs sunny-side up or over easy, cover the pan with a lid and allow the eggs to steam until they are to your liking. If you want them scrambled, gently fold the eggs into the tomato mixture. Remove from heat when the eggs are cooked to the desired consistency. Remove the eggs from the pan and put them into a serving bowl; otherwise the eggs will continue to cook in the heat of the pan.

SPRINKLE with cilantro and serve.

39 grams protein

12 grams net carbs (2 grams fiber)

44 grams total fat

(Nutritional content for full recipe)

Quick Variation

DO you have a favorite fresh salsa? You can use that, or any other salsa you have as long as it's low in sugar. A fresh organic salsa from your deli case could be a great choice. Just heat ½ cup of this salsa in your frying pan and add the eggs for a quick treat.

Power-Packed Pancakes

Serves 2

¾ cup old-fashioned oats or multigrain hot cereal

¼ cup buckwheat flour (Optional. If you don't use this,
add 2 more tablespoons of oats)

¾ cup tofu (or low-fat cottage cheese)

4 egg whites

1 teaspoon vanilla extract

½ teaspoon cinnamon

¼ teaspoon nutmeg

Light cooking-oil spray

MIX the oatmeal, flour (optional), tofu, egg whites, vanilla extract, cinnamon, and nutmeg in a blender until smooth.

SPRAY a nonstick frying pan with cooking spray. Add the batter to the preheated skillet and cook over medium heat until both sides are lightly browned.

TOP the pancake with a no-sugar-added fruit jam. (See the recipe on the next page.)

28 grams protein

41 grams net carbs (7 grams fiber)

7 grams total fat

(Nutritional content for full recipe)

No-Sugar-Added Fruit Jam

6 cups fresh or frozen fruit

1 envelope unflavored gelatin

¾ teaspoon vanilla extract

¼ teaspoon cinnamon

Artificial sweetener to taste (Optional. We don't use any.)

IN a large saucepan over medium heat, bring fruit to a boil. Reduce heat and simmer 35 minutes or until fruit is reduced to 2 cups, stirring occasionally.

IN a small bowl, mix gelatin with vanilla and ¼ cup of the hot fruit, stirring until gelatin is dissolved. Stir mixture into remaining fruit; mix well. Add cinnamon. Cool to nearly room temperature. Stir in sweetener to taste (optional). Cover and refrigerate at least four hours before serving. Store in the refrigerator. Use within two weeks, or freeze and store for up to six months.

7 grams protein

33 grams net carbs (2 grams fiber)

0 grams total fat

(Nutritional content for full recipe)

Variations

MIX different fruits together. Blueberry and plum, strawberry and peach, and mixed berries have all been big successes at our house.

FOR a firmer jam, use two packets of the gelatin.

Spinach Frittata

Serves 2 or 3

THIS recipe fills a 10-inch skillet. If you double the recipe, be sure to use a 14-inch skillet; otherwise, the frittata will be very crispy on the bottom.

6 egg whites

2 egg yolks

¼ cup milk

1 small garlic clove, finely minced

2 green onions, including half of greens, finely sliced

2 tablespoons olive oil

½ large white onion, cut into bite-size cubes

1 crushed garlic clove, finely minced

½ 10-ounce package baby spinach leaves

¼ cup grated or shredded Parmesan or Romano cheese

SET oven on broil. Beat egg whites vigorously until very frothy. Whip in egg yolks and milk. Add garlic and green onions. Set aside.

PREHEAT olive oil in an ovenproof nonstick skillet that can go into the oven. Add white onions and sauté on medium heat until soft. Add garlic and spinach. When spinach has wilted, pour egg mixture over the top, stirring and shaking just enough to make sure the eggs reach the bottom of the pan. Lower heat. Sprinkle Parmesan or Romano over the top.

COOK slowly on low heat until the frittata is firm at the edges and the center is beginning to set. Place under broiler until lightly browned on top. You can serve the frittata either in the pan or on a platter. It will drop in height as it cools.

42 grams protein

45 grams net carbs (7 grams fiber)

15 grams total fat

(Nutritional content for full recipe)

Variations

Spinach and mushroom: Sauté 1 cup sliced mushrooms with onions before adding the spinach.

Spinach and roasted red pepper: Add ½ cup drained, chopped roasted red peppers when adding the spinach.

Ham and cheese: Substitute 1 cup ham for spinach and add 1 cup low-fat cheese when you add the egg mixture.

Mushroom and cheese: Leave out the spinach, sauté 1½ cups mushrooms with onions, and add 1 cup low-fat cheese with the egg mixture.

Spaghetti squash: Substitute 1½ cups steamed spaghetti squash for spinach.

Vinaigrette

¼ cup apple cider vinegar

½ cup extra-virgin olive oil

½ teaspoon dry mustard

Salt and pepper to taste

Artificial sweetener to taste

PUT ingredients into a small mixing bowl or a small container with a tight-fitting lid. Whisk or shake until well mixed. This is enough dressing to last for several meals. Refrigerate after use.

0 grams protein

4 grams net carbs (0 grams fiber)

108 grams total fat

(Nutritional content for full recipe)

Variations

Flavored vinegars: Try different vinegars, such as tarragon, red wine, and balsamic, for a different flavor.

Flavored oils: For a zip, spice up your dressing with jalapeño- or garlic-flavored olive oil. Try different combinations of flavored oils and vinegars. We like balsamic vinegar with the jalapeño oil and some Dijon mustard.

Creamy dressing: Add 2 tablespoons mayonnaise for a creamy dressing. Spice everything up by adding tarragon, thyme, basil, oregano, or other spices of your choice.

Go nuts: Add ¼ cup chopped nuts. One of our favorite dressings is walnut tarragon. Follow the recipe above, substituting tarragon vinegar for the apple cider vinegar. In addition, use 2 tablespoons mayonnaise, 1 teaspoon dried tarragon (or 2 teaspoons fresh), and ¼ cup chopped walnuts.

Four-Bean Chili

Serves 6–8

2 pounds lean beef chuck cut into bite-size pieces,
or 2 pounds lean ground chuck

1 (15.5 oz.) can of each of the following: pinto beans, black
beans, chickpeas, and cannellini beans, drained and rinsed

2 (14.5 oz.) cans diced tomatoes

1 (4 oz.) can chopped green chilies

1 (29 oz.) can crushed tomatoes

1 large onion, chopped

1 tablespoon minced garlic

3 tablespoons chili powder

2 tablespoons ground cumin

2 teaspoons cinnamon

MIX all ingredients in a slow cooker.

COVER and cook on low 8 to 10 hours. If you are using hamburger, stir periodically to break up meat.

THIS is a great recipe for a party because it makes a ton of chili. This hearty chili is good frozen or as leftovers—a great dish for a busy week!

301 grams protein
374 grams net carbs (60 grams fiber)
135 grams total fat
(Nutritional content for full recipe)

Grilled Pork Tenderloin
Serves 6–8

2-pound tenderloin

Asian-style marinade

¼ cup soy sauce

½ cup white wine

¼ cup olive oil

4 green onions, chopped

¼ cup lemon juice

2 cloves garlic, minced

2 tablespoons grated fresh ginger

Ground black pepper to taste

PLACE tenderloin in a flat baking dish or a freezer-proof ziplock bag. Mix all the other ingredients together and pour this marinade over the top of the meat.

MARINATE 18 to 24 hours.

PREHEAT grill, then grill tenderloin over medium flame, reserving marinade.

IF you want to serve extra marinade with the meat, put remaining marinade in a small saucepan, bring to a boil, and allow to boil for at least five minutes.

170 grams protein

0 grams net carbs (0 grams fiber)

50 grams total fat

(Nutritional content for full recipe)

Grilled Vegetables

MANY veggies are excellent grilled. Be experimental and try grilling any of your favorites. Whatever you select, take the clean, dry vegetables and lightly brush them with olive oil or any oil-based marinade. Cooking times will vary, depending on your selection, but most vegetables cook relatively quickly on the grill.

FOR smaller veggies such as snow peas, green beans, bean sprouts, smaller mushrooms (portobellos work great with the above method), simply use a disposable aluminum pie plate, and put in your choice of vegetable, a small amount of olive oil, salt and pepper to taste, and a dash of soy sauce. Wrap the whole thing in aluminum foil and place it on a medium-hot grill. You are essentially steaming the vegetables on the grill. Even Dr. Groll will eat mushrooms this way, and that is saying a whole lot.

Almond-Crusted Chicken
Serves 1–2

Light cooking-oil spray

¾ cup sliced almonds, toasted

2 boneless, skinless chicken breast halves

Salt and pepper to taste

1 egg, beaten

2 tablespoons butter, melted

1 teaspoon lemon juice

1½ teaspoons chopped fresh cilantro

PREHEAT oven to 425°F. Lightly spray baking sheet with cooking oil.

PLACE almonds in a heavy-duty freezer-proof ziplock bag. Lightly crush almonds into small pieces with either your hands or a rolling pin.

GENTLY flatten chicken breasts. Season to taste with salt and pepper.

DIP chicken in beaten egg. Put each chicken breast in bag with almonds; shake until chicken is coated well. Slightly flatten while still in bag. Place chicken on baking sheet. Bake for 10 to 15 minutes or until chicken is just firm and almonds are golden.

MEANWHILE, combine butter, lemon juice, and cilantro. Drizzle over cooked chicken breasts.

76 grams protein

28 grams net carbs (4 grams fiber)

25 grams total fat

(Nutritional content for full recipe)

Orange Salsa

1 cup fresh orange sections (3 oranges) cut into ½-inch pieces

¼ cup minced red onion
(any onion will work, but red or purple onion is prettier)

¼ cup chopped fresh cilantro or mint

¼ teaspoon salt

2 tablespoons lemon juice or 2 teaspoons apple cider vinegar

2 teaspoons minced jalapeño pepper

1 teaspoon olive oil

COMBINE all ingredients in a bowl and stir well. Cover and chill 1 hour.

4 grams protein
50 grams net carbs (10 grams fiber)
15 grams total fat
(Nutritional content for full recipe)

Polynesian Chicken Stir-Fry
Serves 4–6

¼ cup soy sauce

¼ cup sherry

1 teaspoon minced gingerroot

2 garlic cloves, crushed

1 pound boneless, skinless chicken breast, diced

2 tablespoons olive oil

1 medium-size onion

2 cups fresh or frozen bell pepper strips

2 cups chopped fresh pineapple or 1 (20-oz.) can chunk pineapple in light juice, drained

¼ cup sliced almonds (optional)

COMBINE soy sauce, sherry, ginger, and garlic in medium-size bowl and stir well.

ADD chicken. Toss it in the sauce and then marinate in sauce at least 15 minutes.

HEAT olive oil in a large cast-iron skillet or wok. Add chicken and stir-fry until brown and cooked through, about 5 minutes. Remove.

ADD onion, peppers, and pineapple to the skillet; heat through. Pour in sauce and stir. Return chicken to skillet; heat through.

TOP with optional almonds; serve with couscous.

109 grams protein

83 grams net carbs (12 grams fiber)

18 grams total fat

(Nutritional content for full recipe)

Chicken Potpie
Serves 4

Filling

½ cup olive oil

¼ cup whole wheat flour

¼ cup almond meal

1 teaspoon salt

Black pepper to taste

2 tablespoons finely minced onion

2 cups chicken broth

1½ cups sliced mushrooms

3 tablespoons butter

3 cups chopped cooked chicken

2 carrots, chopped

1 medium onion, chopped

2 stalks celery, chopped

Vegan Piecrust (see page 83)

PREHEAT oven to 400°F.

IN a large saucepan, heat olive oil. Blend in flour, almond meal, salt, pepper, and minced onion. Gradually stir in chicken broth. Cook, stirring constantly, until smooth and thickened. In a separate pan, sauté mushrooms in the butter, then stir them into the saucepan. Stir in chicken, carrots, onion, and celery. Mix well and pour into bottom piecrust. Cover with top crust, seal edges, and cut away excess dough. Make several small slits in the top to allow steam to escape.

BAKE in the preheated oven for 30 minutes, or until pastry is golden brown and filling is bubbly.

197 grams protein
307 grams net carbs (60 grams fiber)
408 grams total fat
(Nutritional content for full recipe)

Vegan Piecrust

Makes one 8-inch or 9-inch crust

THIS flaky piecrust with its nutty flavor is a great substitute for the traditional white flour piecrust! It has a nice flavor that accents most fruit pies and potpies and won't send your insulin soaring. Just remember to make sure all the ingredients are really cold when you start; otherwise, the crust won't turn out nearly as good. The flour and nut milk or water can go into the fridge. The canola oil or olive oil should be placed in the freezer for 30 minutes to 1 hour before use.

DOUBLE recipe for a two-crust pie.

1½ cups cold whole wheat flour
¼ cup wheat germ
½ cup cold canola oil (for fruit pies) or olive oil (for potpies)
2 to 4 tablespoons cold nut milk or water

STIR the flour and wheat germ together in a medium-size mixing bowl. Drizzle the oil (it will be very thick) over the mix, while gently stirring it in with a fork, until the mixture resembles coarse meal. Stir in nut milk or water, 1 tablespoon at a time, just until the dough holds together.

ROLL dough into a ball, then roll out into a circle about 12 inches in diameter and ⅛ inch thick.

PLACE in an 8- or 9-inch pie plate and use right away.

30 grams protein

137 grams net carbs (25 grams fiber)

122 grams total fat

(Nutritional content for full recipe)

Fajitas
Serves 2–4

Meat (or Shrimp)

You can choose just about any type of meat for this dish. Use the amount necessary for the group you are serving. This recipe will marinate 4 to 5 pounds of meat and works well for pork, shrimp, beef, or chicken.

Marinade

¼ cup lime juice

¼ cup apple juice

¼ cup olive oil

1 teaspoon minced garlic

¾ teaspoon chili powder

1 teaspoon ground cumin

½ teaspoon cinnamon

Black pepper to taste

WHISK all the marinade ingredients together. Put meat in a heavy-duty ziplock bag. Pour marinade over meat. Marinate 8 to 24 hours.

WHEN your grill is hot, drain the marinade off the meat. Cook meat until done to your liking. Remove from heat and let sit 5 minutes. Cut pork, beef, or chicken into strips against the grain. If you prefer, you can also broil or pan-fry your meat.

128 grams protein

0 grams net carbs (0 grams fiber)

64 grams total fat

(Nutritional content for 1 pound of meat)

Onions and Peppers

2 tablespoons olive oil

1 large onion, separated into rings

2 bell peppers (green, red, yellow—your choice), cut into strips

Salt to taste

HEAT olive oil in a cast-iron skillet over medium heat. Add onion and peppers. Stir until wilted, 3 or 4 minutes. Add salt to taste while stirring. Remove from pan and keep warm.

3 grams protein

24 grams net carbs (4 grams fiber)

24 grams total fat

(Nutritional content for full recipe)

SERVE the fajitas with large lettuce leaves or low-carb whole wheat tortillas, shredded cheese, sour cream, shredded lettuce, salsa, and guacamole.

Meatballs in Saffron-Almond Sauce
Serves 6–8

Meatballs

1 pound ground beef

1 pound ground pork

¼ cup almond meal

¼ cup buckwheat

1 clove garlic, minced

3 tablespoons minced onion

2 tablespoons chopped fresh parsley

½ teaspoon salt

Freshly grated nutmeg to taste

1 egg, beaten

⅓ cup olive oil

Sauce

40 almonds, blanched and skinned

10 black peppercorns

½ teaspoon saffron

1 whole clove

½ teaspoon salt

3 tablespoons olive oil

⅔ cup white wine

1 cup beef or chicken stock

Lemon juice

Chopped parsley

Meatballs

COMBINE all the above ingredients, except the olive oil, in a bowl. Knead until mixture is well blended. Form into small balls (about 36).

HEAT olive oil in a cast-iron skillet. Over medium-low heat, fry meatballs until browned on all sides. Remove and drain.

Sauce

TOAST the almonds either in the oven or in a skillet over low heat. Reserve a few almonds for topping.

PUT almonds, peppercorns, saffron, clove, salt, and wine in a blender or food processor and blend to make a smooth paste. Combine this mixture in a large stockpot with the oil and stock. Bring to a boil, then add the fried meatballs. Simmer the meatballs and sauce for 20 minutes to allow the flavors to blend. Remove from heat.

JUST before serving, add a squeeze of lemon juice.

TRANSFER to a platter. Serve sprinkled with chopped parsley and a few slivered almonds.

276 grams protein

72 grams net carbs (25 grams fiber)

347 grams total fat

(Nutritional content for full recipe)

No-Sugar-Added Apple Pie
Serves 6–8

6 cups peeled and sliced tart apples (approximately 4 large apples)

⅓ cup apple juice concentrate

2 tablespoons quick-cooking tapioca

1 tablespoon cinnamon

½ to ¾ cup chopped almonds

1 tablespoon butter

*2 vegan Piecrusts (put one in a 9-inch pie plate;
reserve the other for top crust of pie)*

PREHEAT oven to 425°F.

IN a large bowl, combine apples, apple juice concentrate, tapioca, and cinnamon; let stand for 15 minutes. Stir and pour into piecrust.

SPRINKLE mixture with nuts and dot with butter. Put on top crust and seal the two crusts together. Cut slits in top crust.

BAKE at 425°F for 15 minutes. Reduce heat to 350°F; bake 40 to 50 minutes longer or until apples are tender. Cover edges with foil during the last 15 minutes of cooking if edges are becoming too brown.

LET the pie cool before serving.

70 grams protein

428 grams net carbs (66 grams fiber)

275 grams total fat

(Nutritional content for full recipe)

Shopping Tips

Here are a few things to keep in mind while you shop for groceries. These tips will help to keep you on track.

Shop the Perimeter

When you're in a hurry, shop only at the perimeter of the grocery store. Don't waste your time and tempt yourself by going down unnecessary aisles. Most grocery stores have shelves stocked with carbs all over the place, but the unprocessed whole foods—meat, dairy, and produce—are on the outside perimeter of the store. Grocery store managers know that low-carbers are being given this advice, so they've also taken to stocking low-carb and organic snacks and foods around the perimeter.

Be Prepared

Spontaneity is grand for a vacation, but not so grand for a diet. One of the best ways to keep yourself on track is to do a little research ahead of time about the nutritional contents of your preferred foods, then plan out a few meals before you head to the grocery store.

Or, if you don't mind spending the extra time in the aisles, bring a pad of paper and a pen with you, and write out your calculations while you're shopping. This way, you'll make sure you're planning properly for an even amount of protein and carbs and half the amount of fat in each of your meals and snacks.

You might want to prepare a few simple meals ahead of time to keep in the refrigerator or freezer, too, so that you don't come home famished one day and reach for the closest bag of junk food or a TV dinner because you don't have the patience to cook a proper meal.

Slip-ups happen; we're all human. Just resolve to give this your best effort and to make a habit of following the plan as closely as possible.

Eat and Run

Now that you have the dietary recommendations down, get those sneakers on, because we're about to switch over to the exercise phase of this program and kick-start your metabolism!

Four

Kick-Start
Your Metabolism

*G*ETTING FIT MAKES you more fertile. Simple as that. Exercise improves your insulin sensitivity.

Committing yourself to the food plan is one part of your program, and that alone can help your fertility a great deal. But exercise is also a major component of this program. Thirty minutes a day, five to six days a week, is all it will take for you to know that you're doing the right thing to regulate your insulin levels and increase your chances of having a baby. You can do that.

Diet and exercise work together in a synergistic relationship. In an additive relationship, one plus one equals two. In a synergistic relationship, the total effect is greater than the sum of the individual parts. The two components complement each other and make the effects of each one stronger, meaning that one (diet) plus one (exercise) could equal five times the effect of either one alone. So if you commit yourself wholeheartedly to this program, you know that you'll increase your fertility potential to the greatest extent possible.

What Exercise Does for You

To understand how exercise will increase your fertility, first we'll need to understand what exercise does for the body in general.

Have you ever noticed how tired you feel after spending hours at a desk or computer terminal? That's because your body is craving exercise. Expending brainpower just isn't the same thing as expending physical energy, and our bodies were designed to be physically active.

Until very recently in the United States, people's daily activities were physically demanding. Recent advances in food storage and preservation, automated labor, and high-tech entertainment have changed our normal lifestyle from active to sedentary. We don't even have to walk around the mall to do holiday shopping anymore or go to the post office to buy stamps. I don't know about you, but sometimes it feels inconvenient when I actually have to go and take out my trash. Couldn't I just download a trash can and hit the "delete" key?

When our grandparents told us how they had to walk to school in the snow, uphill both ways, what they were really telling us is that our modern conveniences have changed our lifestyle. There's a lot of evidence to suggest that the trend toward obesity in the United States over the last two decades has more to do with a lack of exercise than with genetic factors or food.

So we know that our bodies have suffered from our sedentary lifestyle, and so has our energy level. Why do we feel better when we are physically active? Because our bodies were designed for activity—it's our fuel—and without it, we'll always feel as if we're running on fumes.

Two Types of Exercise

There are two distinct forms of exercise: aerobic and resistance. Aerobic exercise is any continuous physical activity that uses up oxygen in the blood by repetitively working large muscle groups and increasing the respiratory and heart rates. Aerobic exercises are typically low-impact, endurance-building activities such as swimming, running, and walking.

Then there's resistance exercise, which is more about working your muscles than about breathing more deeply or getting your heart pumping harder. With resistance exercises (usually weight lifting or calisthenics), you exert energy by sustaining a muscle contraction against a weight. When you do push-ups or chin-ups, for example, the weight is your own body weight—that's the resistance force. These exercises improve muscle strength and promote lean body mass.

These two distinct forms of exercise lead to different physiological changes that promote good health and have specific effects on your body's sensitivity to insulin and, thus, your fertility.

Aerobic Exercise

When you do aerobic exercise, you use more oxygen, and there's an increase in your heart rate, cardiac stroke volume, diastolic blood pressure, and pulse pressure. Blood gets diverted away from your visceral organs (like your gastrointestinal tract) and to the active muscle tissues to meet their increased demand for oxygen.

A regular exercise routine offers you a host of health benefits: lower resting heart rate, lower blood pressure, raised cardiac stroke volume, raised basal metabolic rate, lower percentage of body fat, favorable lipid profiles, and greatly improved oxygen delivery to the tissues. In short, these effects all lead to a smoother-running body that uses oxygen more efficiently. Aerobic exercise helps keep your body in good working condition for every activity, whether that's your ability to catch a bus or your—well, your baby-making endurance!

Resistance Exercise

Sometimes patients teach their doctors. That's what happened when I met Bethany, a 30-year-old woman with polycystic ovary syndrome (PCOS), who had trouble with menses, excessive hair growth, and weight control. She had tried diets, aerobics, and even Metformin medication, but there had been little improvement in her symptoms. It wasn't until she added weight training to her aerobic exercise and a low-carb diet that she achieved an improvement. With this regimen, she was able to control all her symptoms. Her progress is what prompted my investigation on the effects of resistance training on insulin sensitivity.

Although resistance exercise doesn't offer the same cardiovascular benefits as aerobic exercise, it does offer similar metabolic effects and some unique health benefits. Your body fat will diminish, and your lipid profiles will improve, but the most notable benefit of resistance exercise is that your lean body mass (muscles) will develop.

One of the dangers of losing weight is that you also tend to lose muscle. A study published in *Diabetes Care* in 2002 compared two groups of volunteers. The first group completed a high-intensity resistance-training program and a weight-reduction diet; the second group went on the diet but did no resistance training. The volunteers in the first group increased their lean body mass by 0.5 kg. (kilogram, about one pound) in three months, while the second group *lost* 0.4 kg. (just less than a pound) of lean body mass in the same time.[1] That's a difference of about two pounds between the groups! If you're overweight, losing weight is great—but you certainly don't want to lose weight from your muscles. How will you pick up your kids if your muscles have turned to mush?

In addition to improved lean body mass, resistance training also leads to improvements in your basal metabolic rate, endurance, and strength. These effects can improve your energy level and your sense of well-being.

But How Will This Get Me Pregnant?

The physiological effects of exercise we're most interested in for your fertility are its effects on insulin resistance. And both aerobic and resistance exercise will improve your insulin sensitivity, thus making you more fertile.

Your skeletal muscle tissue is the most insulin-sensitive tissue in the body. That is, its ability to use glucose for energy is highly dependent on insulin to work properly. Regular use of the muscle tissue improves its ability to respond to insulin efficiently, partly by improving your mitochondrial function.

Mitochondria

First, a little history. We know that insulin sensitivity declines with age. What we didn't know before was why. Health scientists usually decided that it was because our lean body mass tends to decline as we get older. But a recent study conducted at Yale University found that it might have a different cause.

Researchers compared two groups of people: 15 men and women ages 69 to 84, and 13 men and women ages 18 to 39. The younger and older subjects had similar lean body mass and body fat content, but the older subjects had a much worse response to insulin. To explore this difference, the researchers used nuclear magnetic resonance (NMR) spectroscopy to look at the cells in the subjects' muscle tissue. They found that there were far fewer mitochondria in the older subjects' muscle tissue.

Mitochondria are the cell's powerhouses. They're responsible for converting nutrients into energy—and in the older subjects, the mitochondria were 40 percent less active. But the elderly aren't the only ones whose mitochondria are slacking off on the job.

Several other studies have examined the amount of mitochondria in tissues and the rate of mitochondrial function. Scientists now know that people with insulin resistance (for example, people with type 2 diabetes and their children) have up to 30 percent fewer mitochondria than people who don't have insulin resistance. Additionally, people with insulin resistance have a higher amount of intercellular fatty acids, which is a symptom of lower mitochondrial activity. Those fatty acids get in the way of the enzymes that are trying to transport and metabolize glucose.

But just as you can take control to improve your cholesterol or your weight, you can also improve your mitochondrial function, which then improves your insulin sensitivity, which improves your fertility. How? Through combined aerobic and resistance exercise, of course!

How Aerobic Exercise Affects Mitochondria

Insulin resistance in the skeletal muscles is a main symptom of PCOS and type 2 diabetes, and it also occurs frequently in people who are overweight. The insulin stops working as well as it should, and your muscles become less effective at transporting glucose and synthesizing glycogen.

Physical inactivity for even just a couple of days will lead to a rapid decline in oxygen uptake, muscle activity, and mitochondrial activity. But you can actually put a stop to all these negative effects by maintaining a physically active lifestyle.

Aerobic exercise actually increases the mitochondrial surface area and DNA content: that is, the actual number of mitochondria increases. As you exercise regularly, your body will also get better at using oxygen and energy, and you'll "toughen up" to minimize muscle damage, so that your exercise capacity will be greater and greater as you go along. What feels hard today might feel easy in just a couple of months because you've built up your body's ability to withstand strain.

Also, as you exercise, more taxi drivers will want to work for you. Huh?

GLUT-4 is a protein that transports glucose into skeletal muscle cells. Glucose has a hard time getting past the bouncers (the cell membranes), so GLUT-4, a friendly taxi driver, helps it along. Glucose gets into the cab, and GLUT-4 drives right through the cell membrane and into the muscle cell (and doesn't even play bad music in the car).

If you sit and watch talk shows all day, your taxi drivers go on strike. They decide to sit next to you and eat snack cakes, too, instead of doing their job of getting glucose into the muscles. Free fatty acids crash the party in the muscle cells. They have a grand time playing tricks on your insulin levels and keeping the muscle cells nice and crowded so that the GLUT-4 doesn't come back. The glucose just hangs out outside the cell entrance, trying to persuade the tough bouncer membranes to let it in, before giving up and going back to the bloodstream.

Guess what happens then? Call out the insulin!

Insulin can't stand seeing stragglers hanging out in the wrong place, so it comes rushing out to clear the glucose out of the blood. This could all be stopped if only the mitochondria were functioning better. Mitochondria have the power to toss out the free fatty acids, preventing these acids from crowding out the taxi drivers. Then the taxi drivers could take the glucose into the party where it belongs, and the insulin wouldn't have to work itself into a frenzy trying to play "clean up the streets."

You, dear woman, have the ability to empower those mitochondria. All you have to do is get into a regular routine of aerobic exercise, and your mitochondria won't disappear, your taxi drivers won't go on strike, and your insulin can stay calm and regulated.

How Resistance Exercise Helps

It's true that the improvement in mitochondrial function seen with aerobic exercise is generally not seen with resistance training. However, resistance training does lead to increased muscle mass. It also helps your body move and use glucose more smoothly, and this effect ultimately leads to a better capacity to exercise. You'll have more strength and better oxygen delivery, which will make it easier for you to build your stamina for future workouts.

Here's the Proof

Basic scientific theory can help us understand the very complicated processes within our bodies, but until we have clinical data showing us how exercise has helped real people, we're just guessing about the effects. Luckily, in the last several years a series of clinical studies has demonstrated the profound impact that exercise has on improving insulin sensitivity.

Four studies in particular tested the role of exercise in preventing diabetes. These studies enrolled between 500 and 3,000 glucose-intolerant men and women of various ethnic backgrounds and ages, all of whom were insulin-resistant. In all the studies, the participants were put on an aerobic exercise regimen, and two of the studies included resistance training. In every study, the participants demonstrated significant reductions in developing diabetes, and improved insulin sensitivity.

When evaluating resistance exercise, researchers found that participants showed more improvement in insulin sensitivity than with aerobic exercise alone. When resistance exercise was added to aerobic programs, the participants showed 25 percent less insulin resistance and almost three times more glucose delivery to the tissues by insulin. When resistance training was eliminated from the exercise regimen for as little as 90 days, the participants showed a 33 percent drop in insulin-mediated glucose disposal.

Given this information, we know that if we want to minimize the bad effects of insulin on your fertility, we need to combine an insulin-lowering diet program with an exercise regimen containing both aerobic and resistance exercise.

Ready for My Push-Ups, Mr. DeMille

Before we get into the specifics of the exercise program, a warning is in order. People with underlying medical problems can get hurt by jumping into a new exercise regimen. Anyone who has unstable angina, uncontrolled blood pressure (systolic greater than 160 mm [millimeters] Hg or diastolic greater than 100 mm Hg, or both), heart irregularities, congestive heart failure, almost any heart valve problems, or cardiomyopathy should not participate in this exercise regimen. If you have any concern regarding any other medical problems or injuries, please consult your doctor before starting this program. That said, crank up the music and let's get moving.

The basis for our exercise recommendations comes from the Diabetes Prevention Program, a study of more than 3,000 people with insulin resistance. It's the largest study of its kind, and over the course of four years it found a 59 percent reduction in cases of type 2 diabetes through lifestyle intervention. Because insulin resistance (which is at the heart of our concerns about infertility) is so closely linked with type 2 diabetes, the study is very applicable to our needs.

Goals of Aerobic Exercise

YOUR GOAL

Aerobic exercise for 30 minutes a day, 5 or 6 days per week.

ACCEPTABLE EXERCISES

Walking, jogging, swimming, cycling, gardening.

EXERCISE GOAL

50 to 60 percent rise in heart rate from baseline.

The participants in the Diabetes Prevention Program did low-impact aerobic exercise (usually walking) for 150 minutes per week. To make this a regular part of your daily routine—which gives you a much better shot at keeping up with it on a long-term basis—we recommend breaking it up into 30-minute workouts five days per week. You can do whatever kind of aerobic exercise you like as long as you're raising your heart rate by 50 to 60 percent of your baseline heart rate throughout your exercise. First, you need to check your pulse before you begin exercising. If you have a resting heart rate of 80 beats per minute, then 50 percent of that is 40 beats per minute, so your target heart rate would be 80 plus 40: about 120 beats per minute.

You don't want to just shock your body into action, though. Remember that every good aerobic workout has a cycle: warm-up, peak, maintaining your target heart rate, then cooling down with stretches. The first five minutes or so of your workout should consist of light-intensity actions such as walking, cycling, or an easy jog as a warm-up. The fitness trainer Jon Freeman says that at the peak of your workout you should aim to sustain a sprint pace for 5 to 10 minutes—make it as intense as you can without feeling like you're going to collapse. Then, instead of stopping and lying down on the floor after you're through, make sure you spend at least another five minutes slowing down your pace, possibly walking again, then stretching your muscles thoroughly to avoid getting cramps and injuries.

Goals of Resistance Exercise

> **YOUR GOAL**
>
> *Include a resistance or strengthening workout*
> *2 or 3 times per week.*
>
> **ACCEPTABLE EXERCISES**
>
> *Bench presses, push-ups, pull-ups, biceps curls, leg presses,*
> *quadriceps curls, toe raises, rowing, water aerobics.*
>
> **EXERCISE GOALS**
>
> *If you're using weights, find the maximum weight you can handle.*
> *Then do one set of 8 to 12 exercises using 40 to 60 percent*
> *of that weight for each of the exercises.*

For resistance training, include a single set of eight to twelve different exercises, focusing on the major muscle groups, performed two or three times per week. Examples of resistance exercises include chest presses, shoulder presses, triceps extensions, biceps curls, pull-downs (upper back), lower-back extensions, abdominal crunches, quadriceps extensions, leg presses, and leg curls (for hamstrings).

You can perform these exercises in a variety of ways, such as through calisthenics, free weights, pulley weight machines, or rubber band resistance machines. All of these can be effective, so the important part is to find a method you are comfortable with.

In terms of how much weight to use, you should base your training on your one-repetition maximum (RM). Your RM is the most resistance you can meet to perform one repetition of a given exercise—for example, how much you can bench-press if you have to do it only a single time.

When you're just starting out, you should use a resistance of approximately 40 percent of your RM, so you won't injure your muscles and burn yourself out. If your RM on a particular exercise is 100 pounds, you'll want to do a set of repetitions of that exercise using a weight of 40 pounds. As you gain practice and time, you can build up to about 60 percent of your RM for a typical workout, so you'll do those 8 to 10 repetitions using 60 pounds of weight.

So, you may be wondering, how many repetitions are in a set? As many as you can handle.

When you work out, I want you to keep going on each exercise until you experience volitional fatigue—a term that means "I can't lift this anymore!" One set done in this fashion has the same strengthening effects as a multiple-set regimen using fewer repetitions, so this will keep your workouts efficient and effective.

When planning your workout, try to exercise opposite muscle groups in the same workout session. For example, if you're working your chest or biceps, also include back or triceps exercises. This keeps your strengthening balanced and reduces your risk of injury.

You don't need to exercise every muscle group every time you do resistance exercise. You might focus on your calves and thighs during one session, on your chest and back during another session, and on your glutes and arms during the next session. It's hard to tire out your abdominal muscles, though, so doing crunches every session is a good idea! And just as with aerobics, you need to take time to stretch at the end of your resistance workout. Many gyms offer a free introductory session in which a trainer will teach you proper workout techniques and methods for stretching.

Add Water and Watch Your Muscles Grow

Water aerobics combine the best of both exercise worlds. You can get all the health benefits of aerobics, and at the same time, the water provides the resistance needed for resistance exercises.

This kind of exercise is especially good for those who have any injuries, arthritis, or back problems, and has long been used as a form of physical therapy because it's relaxing and easy on the joints, carrying almost no risk of injury to muscles, bones, or joints. It's a gentle way to increase muscle strength and reach your target heart rate at the same time.

You don't even have to know how to swim, and you don't need to submerge yourself underwater like the Olympic water ballet team. Typically, you'll work out in chest-deep warm (not hot) water, and you can do most of the same aerobic exercises that you would do on land. You'll just do them more slowly.

If you've ever tried to run in a pool, you'll know that feeling of running in slow-motion. That's because water offers 12 times as much resistance as air. But even though it's harder to move, you'll probably feel less strained after a water workout than you would after a land workout. And you can reap all the same benefits as the landlubbers.

Check to see if your local gym, YMCA, or pool offers a class. If not, you can just take your normal aerobic routine and submerge it! You can also find a large pool and try to "speed-walk" your way around it several times. No special gear is needed, but you can buy weights that are specifically meant for water exercises, if you like, and you'll probably want a pair of aqua shoes (available at most department stores) for traction. Remember that even if you don't feel you're working out as strenuously, you still need to warm up before you start and cool down with stretches afterward.

Yoga

You don't need to put on a tank top and stand next to the bulked-up guys with barbells at the gym to get your resistance exercise. Hatha yoga is an excellent way to get resistance training and possibly help you feel more relaxed and grounded, too.

Yoga isn't just about contorting your body into weird positions. It's about stretching, strengthening, toning, meditating, breathing, and releasing tension. Yoga has a spiritual basis, but it's up to you how you want to use it. Whether or not you believe it can help you tap into the "universal consciousness" and live in harmony with nature, the physical act of practicing yoga postures (known as asanas) will help you meet your exercise goals to increase your fertility.

Yoga has several benefits. First, you can do it anywhere. If you're stuck at your desk and you have just a ten-minute break, you don't even have to stand up. There are several postures you can practice while seated. Second, it leaves plenty of room for progress. There are a wide variety of "beginner" postures that nearly anyone can do, and once you're ready to move on, you can try increasingly harder poses. Third, there's a low possibility of injury (this is why, like water aerobics, yoga is often recommended to people with medical concerns).

You can take a class or buy a yoga video or DVD; you may even find one at your local library to borrow. Wear loose clothes, pick up an exercise mat, and go barefoot if you like.

Pilates

You've doubtless heard about Pilates lately, thanks to the fact that seemingly every celebrity in Hollywood from Joan Collins to Sharon Stone has discovered its benefits. But Pilates is no recent trend; it was actually developed in the 1920s, though it never received much publicity until about 10 years ago.

Dancers were among the first to take an interest in Pilates, because it's designed to help build long, lean muscles without adding bulk, and it's associated with improved balance and flexibility. It also concentrates a great deal on strengthening abdominal and back muscles, generally referred to as the body's "core." The resistance is good not only for improving insulin sensitivity but also for strengthening bones.

There are hundreds of exercises in the Pilates program, and one of the key principles is to stress control and precision. Because of this, Pilates instructors encourage quality over quantity: precise movements in excellent posture rather than many repetitions until you're exhausted.

As with yoga, all you really need is a mat, and you don't need to be in great shape to start. Pilates is appropriate for people of all ages and all degrees of athletic skill. There's more variety of exercises available if you use specially designed Pilates equipment, which you can find at gyms or buy for home use. A fitness ball costs about $12 in department stores and can add diversity to your routine.

Both Pilates and yoga are "total body" workout systems. You don't choose just a few muscle groups and build them. You work several muscle groups at once, and each workout should be done in a particular order.

If you discover that you love Pilates, there are even "prenatal Pilates" tapes showing exercises that are safe to do during pregnancy.

Nia

If you're looking for a social outlet to go with your exercise, you might try Neuromuscular Integrative Action, or Nia. It's a form of "fusion fitness," because it combines more than one classic movement form. It incorporates exercises from martial arts, healing arts, and dance, and it's a nonimpact program that won't stress your knees or shins.

On their website, Nia's creators, Debbie and Carlos Rosas, write, "Nia fully supports the pleasure principle: If it feels good, keep doing it. If it hurts, stop!"

They believe that the militaristic element often found in typical fitness classes is actually harmful because it creates "resistance and insecurity, rather than enthusiasm and self-respect."

Nia works for the aerobic portion of your exercise goals, and it encourages playfulness, body awareness, and freedom of expression. In this environment, you'll often find a sense of community among the participants. There are also retreats, camps, and workshops throughout the United States and many other countries.

To learn more about Nia and find classes near you, visit the Nia Technique website at www.nia-nia.com.

Rowing

Rowing machines also provide both aerobic and resistance exercise. In addition, rowing can help you strengthen bones in the axial skeleton (your spine and hips), which is the most common place for osteoporotic fractures. If you row quickly, you get more of an aerobic workout. If you choose more resistance and row slowly, you're getting more of a strength workout. Of course, if you have access to a boat and a couple of oars, this exercise is just as good on an open lake!

Never Say Never!

Maybe you've never thought of yourself as a jock. Maybe you think all this stuff about exercise is intimidating. Let me tell you about Charlotte.

When she became my patient, Charlotte was a 36-year-old with two prior successful pregnancies. But she had continually gained weight, especially after her second pregnancy, and she was now up to 210 pounds. Her weight was mostly distributed around her midsection, consistent with symptoms of insulin resistance. Her menstrual cycles became more irregular and bothersome, and despite not using contraception from the time of her last pregnancy, she had not conceived in three years.

She started her lifestyle program with both diet and exercise, and within three months she reestablished a regular cycle. On the fourth cycle, surprise! With her improved menstrual cycle also came improved fertility, and her third son was conceived.

Now for the fun part. Since that third pregnancy, she has been able to keep her weight down, and the formerly overweight mother of three got so good at building stamina and strength in her new exercise lifestyle that she has just completed her first half marathon!

Want to be like Charlotte?

Start now. Not tomorrow or next week. Make time to get that body moving today.

Sample Workout Regimens

Schedule 1

Monday: Low-impact aerobics or water aerobics class for 30 minutes.

Tuesday: Walk at a brisk pace for 30 minutes. Upper-body resistance: biceps curls, triceps extensions, chest presses, latissimus (back) pulls, trapezoid lifts, abdominal crunches.

Wednesday: Walk for 30 minutes.

Thursday: Rest.

Friday: Pilates for 30 minutes.

Saturday: Swim for 30 minutes. Lower-body resistance: toe raises (calf), quad extensions, chest presses, hamstring curls, leg presses (squats), leg adductions, leg abductions, abdominal crunches.

Sunday: Rest.

Schedule 2

Monday: Yoga for 30 minutes. Walk at a brisk pace for 30 minutes.

Tuesday: Cycle for 30 minutes.

Wednesday: Rest.

Thursday: Walk for 30 minutes.

Friday: Dance for 30 minutes. Use Nautilus or Bowflex machine for 20 minutes.

Saturday: Rest.

Sunday: Jog for 30 minutes.

Of course, you can substitute any applicable type of exercise—the point is just to get some aerobic exercise five times a week and resistance training at least twice a week.

As an alternative, you can do circuit training. There are specialized gyms such as Curves (with locations all over the country) that design 30-minute workouts combining both aerobic and resistance exercises on a timed schedule. Curves is a women-only gym, and you move from station to station in time with music, so you don't have to stand around and wait to use a particular machine. Many women prefer the atmosphere at an all-women gym like this, saying there's less pressure to look like a supermodel and there's a more friendly (less show-offish) environment. To learn more and check for locations, visit www.curvesinternational.com.

Or try these similar fitness centers that also offer circuit training:

• Liberty Fitness Center: www.libertyfitness.com
• Contours Express: www.contoursexpress.com
• Slim and Tone: www.slimandtone.com

Keep It Up

You now have the foundation of our program: the meal plan and the exercise plan. Together, these are the best tools you have to get your insulin on track and take control of your fertility. But starting is one thing and staying on track is another. For this program to work for you, you need to commit to it—starting right now! In Chapter 5, we'll discuss ways for you to keep yourself motivated to stick to your goals.

Five

Planning for Success

F OR ANY PROGRAM to work, you have to see it through. Believing in your dream is one thing; committing yourself to its fruition is another. Nearly all of us have tried diet and exercise programs and failed. Often it's because we just didn't keep up with them as we expected to in the beginning. So how can we improve the likelihood that this time will be any different?

Setting Goals

We all have dreams. Dreams are the visions we have of our ideal life: things we'd like to accomplish, things we'd like to own, honors we'd like to earn. Goals help us get those dreams out of our head and into our reality. Actively setting goals makes it more likely that you will achieve your dreams.

Goals help you define where you want to commit your time and energy, as well as what's not so important. In this way, they provide a road map for your actions.

A healthy pregnancy depends on many factors, some of which are out of your control. So while your larger goal may be to have a healthy baby, I want you to focus on setting tangible goals that you can measure and accomplish. You can set goals such as eating a certain amount of protein in a day, or exercising for a particular amount of time per day, but you shouldn't make your goal "Get pregnant by next month." That can make you feel like a failure even if you're doing everything right and even if your body is responding well to your efforts.

How to Set Goals

Setting goals is a learned skill, not an instinct. There are certain guidelines you can follow to make your goals most effective and most achievable.

Write Down Your Goals!

Most important, you must write down your goals. The simple act of placing something on paper raises your level of commitment. It just feels different: it's no longer an ethereal dream, but a concrete plan of action that you intend to follow.

Written materials provide tangible reminders of the bigger picture. They'll help you keep focused. Studies have found that if you don't write down your goals, you have a 3 to 7 percent chance of achieving them, whereas if you do write them down, you have a 70 to 80 percent chance of success. That's a tremendous difference!

Make Active Statements

Write your goals as active statements starting with the word "to." For example, "To exercise 30 minutes per day five days per week." This makes the goal a specific target that requires your action to accomplish it.

Set Deadlines

Goals need dates and times. Be honest now: When did you write your school reports? The day before they were due? When do you file your taxes? After April 10?

There's a big difference between "someday" and "tomorrow." If your boss said to you, "I'd like you to fill out this paperwork eventually, whenever you have a chance," you'd probably put it on your desk, where it would be forgotten under a pile of sticky notes and mail until the boss mentioned it again. If, however, the boss said, "Please have this paperwork on my desk by tomorrow morning," you'd get to it right away.

So it goes with setting goals. We're deadline-driven people, and a deadline helps us to give ourselves timelines for progress. If you don't reach your goal by the specified time, set a new deadline! Don't leave it up to chance. Write down a new deadline, and don't stop until you've reached your goal.

Identify Obstacles

The natural response to setting a date is to ask, "How will I get this done in time?" In fact, it's good to have a few doubts, because they'll let you be realistic about the obstacles that may stand in your way. There will always be obstacles in the path toward any goal; what's important is how you overcome them. It's best to think about obstacles in advance rather than wait for them to pop up when you're too busy to figure out what to do about them.

For every obstacle you can think of, write down an action that will help you move past it. Let's say that your goal is to meet the daily protein requirement each day within four weeks. Here are a few examples of obstacles that may come up and active solutions you can use:

- Obstacle: I don't like eggs or meat for breakfast.
  Action: I will try making fruit smoothies for breakfast and adding protein powder to them.
- Obstacle: I'm frequently on the road at lunchtime, and I often eat fast food.
  Action: I will keep protein bars or meal replacement bars in my glove compartment so I'm not tempted to stop at fast-food places.
- Obstacle: My grocery bill may be higher.
  Action: I will reallocate some of our entertainment budget to the grocery budget.

Check Your Progress

When you're first setting your goals, you may not anticipate all the obstacles, or you may find the opposite: that a goal was easier than you expected and you can move on to more difficult goals.

Likewise, life continually evolves, and you may find that your goals will need to be updated from time to time to suit your current needs. Modify your goals as necessary.

Remember that setting goals is a means to an end: reaching your dreams. When achieving your goals seems difficult, remind yourself of the big picture and what you're striving for.

Make Your Journal a Joy

It's a fact—recording your daily efforts to meet your goals will give you a better chance of achieving them. Keeping a journal is one of the least expensive and most effective ways of improving your results with our program.

Researchers at the University of Maryland put 50 obese women on a weight-loss program for six months and studied the results to determine what behaviors made the women either successful or unsuccessful at losing weight. Do you want to know what the number one factor was in determining who lost weight and who didn't? The ones who carefully wrote down the type and amount of food they ate were the ones who succeeded. Maintaining a weight graph also helped.[1]

Another study, conducted by researchers at Albert Einstein College of Medicine, put this experiment into an even more modern setting. They watched 588 people on a weight-loss diet to see who would lose the most weight. They, too, found that people who kept a daily workbook lost weight. But people who wrote in their workbooks and also used a computer-assisted journal program lost more than twice as much weight! So if you're technologically inclined, you might want to commit yourself to checking in with your keyboard once a day, too.[2]

This is what worked for Lynette Peters, a 28-year-old woman from New Jersey who says that keeping a food log is one of the most important parts of her low-carb lifestyle.

"I keep track of everything I eat, on a website called Fitday.com," she says. "It adds up the calories, fat, carbs, and protein in my daily intake and really helps me keep track of what I put into my mouth. Plus, it's great for helping you to watch what you eat if you know that you'll have to input it later and actually 'see' it."

Researchers at OSF-St. Francis Medical Center wanted to find out whether self-monitoring could stop people from putting on pounds during the toughest time of all: the holidays. They found that people in the study tended to gain 500 percent more weight during holiday weeks than during other weeks and that the only people in the study who lost weight during the 10 weeks the study lasted were the ones who were most consistent with self-monitoring—that is, writing down everything they ate.[3]

Now, these studies all had to do with weight loss, which isn't necessarily the goal of our program. However, the results are applicable to our program. Whether it's a weight-loss diet or a fertility program, what these researchers found is that people who wrote down everything they did in relation to the program were the ones who succeeded. Weight loss is easy to measure in clinical trials. But even if you're not trying to lose weight, you can safely assume that keeping a daily journal of your food intake and your progress in exercise will improve your outcome.

Why a Journal Works

A journal helps us for at least three reasons: it gives us a clearer picture of reality, it makes us accountable for our actions, and it establishes a routine for us.

DID I REALLY EAT THAT?

Sometimes when we look back on our day, we remember the major meals, but we forget the little snacks we ate while driving, watching television, or even while cooking. Or we forget that we went back for seconds, ate a double portion of pasta, or noshed on fried appetizers while waiting for the main course at a restaurant.

The same goes for time management. It's pretty easy to convince yourself that you have no time to exercise—after all, you're the busiest person on the planet.

Before you begin your program, why not try this experiment for yourself? Every half hour for a day or two, take just a few seconds to jot down what you're doing. See when you're really just "wasting time" and when you could claim more time to do the things you really want to do.

Some of the most likely time bandits are television, beauty rituals, e-mail, Web browsing, shopping, and cleaning.

Try completing this chart two days in a row and see what you come up with.

ACTIVITIES CHART

Time	Activity	Time	Activity
12:00 midnight		12:00 noon	
12:30 a.m.		12:30 p.m.	
1:00 a.m.		1:00 p.m.	
1:30 a.m.		1:30 p.m.	
2:00 a.m.		2:00 p.m.	
2:30 a.m.		2:30 p.m.	
3:00 a.m.		3:00 p.m.	
3:30 a.m.		3:30 p.m.	
4:00 a.m.		4:00 p.m.	
4:30 a.m.		4:30 p.m.	
5:00 a.m.		5:00 p.m.	
5:30 a.m.		5:30 p.m.	
6:00 a.m.		6:00 p.m.	
6:30 a.m.		6:30 p.m.	
7:00 a.m.		7:00 p.m.	
7:30 a.m.		7:30 p.m.	
8:00 a.m.		8:00 p.m.	
8:30 a.m.		8:30 p.m.	
9:00 a.m.		9:00 p.m.	
9:30 a.m.		9:30 p.m.	
10:00 a.m.		10:00 p.m.	
10:30 a.m.		10:30 p.m.	
11:00 a.m.		11:00 p.m.	
11:30 a.m.		11:30 p.m.	

Before you start feeling guilty, let's first assert that if you find joy in a particular leisure-time activity, you don't need to quit doing it. If you love watching *American Idol,* we're not trying to tell you that you should be exercising during the time it's on. What we are suggesting is that you limit your time bandits to the ones that really matter to you.

As network executives know, a large percentage of people will keep the television on after their favorite show has ended. That's how we wind up watching shows we never intended to watch—maybe even shows we don't really like. They're just sort of on, and we never turned the television off, so we're passively sitting there on the couch, forgetting that we have the option to do other things.

So by all means, if you have a favorite show, or time set aside to read or check your e-mail, don't feel guilty about it. Be aware, however, of how much "extra" time is tagging along in the process. Or if you think your mornings are full and by the time you get home at night you're too tired to exercise, why not see how you could juggle things to free half an hour every morning? Try moving the less strenuous activities to later in the day so you can get your body moving as early as possible.

By taking a look at your Activities Chart, you can figure out where you could curtail your "extraneous" activities and make some time to exercise. Note that I did say "make some time." That's a big difference between people who get things done and people who don't. One group says, "I don't have time." The other says, "I will make time."

Join the second group. Figure out where you could fit in 30 minutes of exercise five or six times a week. Experiment until you "make" the right time for you.

ACCOUNTABILITY

You might be surprised by how much the thought of having to write down a poor choice of food in your journal is a deterrent to eating it. When you are in the routine of writing down everything that goes into your mouth, it will become automatic to think about writing down any foods before you eat them. White bread, soda, and potato chips suddenly seem less appealing when you know they're going to be showcased in writing and serve as a mark against your progress.

In any program, it helps to be accountable to someone. When you keep a journal, you're becoming accountable to yourself. You're serving as the monitor of your own progress, and you'll judge your own performance on the basis of the evidence in your journal.

Bigger Is Better

In the case of journals, size does matter.

Go for a full notebook-size journal. It doesn't have to be a fancy one from a stationery store; you can find a planner at an office supply store, or even use a typical three-ring binder with loose-leaf paper, a marbled notebook, or a legal pad. This way it's harder to lose or overlook.

Keep It Visible

Keep your journal out in an obvious spot, preferably in the kitchen so it's easiest to get to right after a meal. Don't stick it in a drawer or under a pile of papers—leave it right out on the kitchen counter or table, even if company is coming.

The more you can do to make your journal visible and handy, the better chance you have of using it regularly. Try to leave it in the same spot all the time, so that you know exactly where it is and so that reaching for it several times a day becomes an instinct.

Several Times a Day?

Yes, that's right. Many people think it's okay to leave a journal on their nightstand and write everything in it just once a day: before they go to bed. But this system relies on your having an outstanding memory.

By the time you go to bed, do you really remember everything you ate and in what portions? Could you really remember the number of grams of carbs in your sandwich?

Ideally, you want to write in your journal right after every meal and snack. You might want to keep a small notebook in your pocket-book so you can jot down notes about your meals, your snacks on the go, and your time at the gym, then transfer them into your journal once you get home.

Make It Yours

What will encourage you to use your journal? How can you make it physically attractive to increase its psychological appeal?

The goal is to make this journal something you'll want to look at, pick up, and use frequently. If you know you have a tendency to forget, you might want to choose a fluorescent pink or yellow notebook, so it's practically glowing. If you value beauty, make your journal beautiful. Either choose one that catches your fancy or decorate a plain one yourself, any way you please, with glitter, lace, markers, photos, or any other craft material you care to use.

Reward Yourself

If you have trouble getting started or committing yourself to writing in your journal, set rewards for yourself.

A trip to Bermuda would be a nice reward, of course, but perhaps just a little impractical. Think smaller. For example, if you love that morning cup of coffee, don't let yourself have it until you've written in your journal. If there's a television show you can't do without, don't turn it on until the journal is up to date.

And it is important to apply the same kinds of rewards to the program itself. How can you find ways to treat yourself when you've met all your exercise goals for the week? How can you reward yourself for dutifully reading labels and making smart meal choices?

Choose something that brings you joy, whether it's talking on the phone with your sister, going bowling, or getting a pedicure.

What Do I Write?

The bare minimum to write down is all *(all!)* your food choices and all your exercise efforts each day. Even if you had just three bites of that chocolate cake, you must write them down and analyze their nutritional content.

Here's a sample worksheet to show you what's required. You may certainly have more food than the number of slots here; this is just an example.

DAILY MEAL PLAN WORKSHEET

Daily Nutritional Needs

Protein =   Carbs =   Fat =

Food Choice	Protein grams	Carb grams	Fat grams
Breakfast:			
Morning snack:			
Lunch:			
Dinner:			
Bedtime snack:			
Daily nutritional intake (add the columns)			

Then, track your exercise every day. If you did nothing on a certain day, force yourself to note that, too. Big zeroes or sad faces all over your chart aren't pleasant to look at. Maybe seeing them will be a deterrent to neglecting your exercise.

EXERCISE WORKSHEET

Exercise goal: 30 minutes of aerobic exercise 5 or 6 times per week; 15 to 20 minutes of resistance exercise or 8 to 12 resistance exercises 2 or 3 times per week

Day of Week	Aerobic Exercise	Time Spent	Resistance Exercise	Time Spent
Monday				
Tuesday				
Wednesday				
Thursday				
Friday				
Saturday				
Sunday				

At the end of the day, review your journal. Whether you met all your goals for the day or your willpower wavered, write down at least one good thing you did for yourself in terms of your fertility lifestyle program. You may want to take notes about your progress—for example, you might write a quick line about days when you were able to increase your weight in resistance exercises, or put stars next to the days when you met all your food goals for the day.

You could take notes about how you felt each day, which may give you a barometer to show you how you're progressing. You may begin the first few exercise sessions feeling weak and tired but then notice, as the weeks go on, that your energy level and mood improve. At first, you may find it frustrating and difficult to get used to reading labels and analyzing your food, but soon these habits become second nature and you barely have to glance at labels to know what's a good choice and what isn't.

The fact that you've written something down helps you commit it to memory, so keeping a daily food journal will make it easier to get to know the nutritional values of your favorite foods. This way, you won't have to stop and question yourself every time you want a snack; and mixing and matching recipes will become easy.

This is your journal, and no one's going to grade it, so feel free to doodle in the margins, write in bubble letters, give yourself stickers, or do anything else that will make it enjoyable for you to record your efforts.

Be Kind

Kids lie when they think the truth will be unacceptable. They say they have no idea who broke the vase because they think you might love them less if they own up to their mistake.

Adults do the same thing, though in a more subtle manner. The worst, though, is when we lie to ourselves.

You may be tempted to leave out some of your food choices, or to claim you got your aerobic exercise for the day because you walked up and down the stairs a few times to put away the laundry. But really, you're only hurting yourself.

Don't expect perfection from yourself. The object of keeping this journal is not to be an A+ student. What you're trying to achieve here is a pattern. On an average day, how well are you meeting your goals for food and exercise? What areas need improvement? When do you tend to fall short of your goals? What can you do to fix shortfalls?

Remember that this isn't a "sometimes" program. For the program to work, in terms of your fertility, you need to maintain it on a regular basis. It does you no good to keep your insulin levels in check for a day or two, then send them spiking through the roof because you feel that you have "been good" and that now you can take a day off from the program.

A piece of cake once a week won't derail your efforts. Junk food every night, starchy food several times a week, or a total lack of regular exercise will.

Kisha Washington came to my clinic when she was 30 years old. She already had two children but now had been trying for another child for more than a year without success. To complicate matters, she had PCOS and had developed type 2 diabetes.

She was taking 1,000 mg. per day of Metformin and monitoring her diet to treat her diabetes, and she was in good control with regard to glucose. But when we are considering pregnancy, we try to get hemoglobin A1c (a marker of long-term sugar control) below 6 percent. Hers was 6.2 percent. So I gave her my recommendations for diet and exercise.

It was hard to reduce her carbs, she says. "Sometimes I slipped, but I just had to get back up and start over. Some days, you pass that doughnut shop, and, *Oh, God!* I was a junk food eater. I love chips and I love cookies. It was really hard to give up my cookies, but I had to do what I had to do to get pregnant. If I ate carbs, it was whole-grain carbs. Brown rice was the most awful thing I had ever tasted, but I got used to it!"

Within one month, she brought her A1c down to 5.8 percent and had dropped from size 16 to 14. She had already been bicycling and walking, but she added resistance training to her regimen, and she feels that this made the big difference for her. Before that, she says she was losing weight, but it wasn't until she started lifting weights that she felt her body had changed for the better.

"I really think weight training is good—nothing excessive; you don't have to get big muscles, but just try to keep yourself toned," she says.

She conceived during her second month of following my program without any fertility medications. Now she says she's maintaining the health habit—she has continued to cycle and lift light weights during her pregnancy, and now that she knows what to eat and is used to eating vegetables instead of junk food, she plans to keep doing so. Does she give in to temptation every now and then? Sure, but she's careful to pay attention to her everyday habits, just as she did when she was trying to conceive. She kept her overall goal in mind and succeeded.

So observe your patterns, and don't beat yourself up for minor transgressions. If you're kind to yourself and accepting of your results, you'll be more likely to be honest with yourself and write down your true daily food choices and exercise efforts. Don't avoid or "purposely forget" to write in your journal on days when you haven't met your goals. It's important to write everything down, good and bad.

You may find a tremendous sense of accomplishment when you see how well you're doing, or how you're improving. Even if you're still falling short of some goals each week, try your best to get closer and closer to the goal as time goes on. It may take you a few weeks to build up to total compliance with the program, and that's okay. Be kind to yourself as you make these efforts; lifestyle changes can take a little while to "stick," especially if they run counter to the habits you've formed your whole life.

Let your journal help you gain perspective on how you're doing, and you'll have your own built-in fertility progress report.

Emotional Support

*t*HE GOAL OF any therapy is to improve the quality of life for the person undergoing it. Improved quality of life may mean achieving a pregnancy, but it also means easing the emotional stress for those who haven't yet or ultimately won't become pregnant.

The Emotional Scene

In clinical tests, physiological measurements of stress response hormones haven't been significantly higher in infertile patients than in control subjects. Numerous studies have found that stress plays, at most, a very minor role in infertility. However, infertile patients tend to have extremely high scores on stress inventories: questionnaires in which patients check off stressful events and symptoms in their lives and are scored on the basis of the items they check. Also, clinical depression is very common among women who have actively tried to achieve a pregnancy for two years and haven't been successful.

Women who have problems with fertility will often experience depressed moods, anxiety, problems with sleep, "stress eating," feelings of hopelessness, feelings of helplessness, constant worrying about why they are not getting pregnant or whether they will ever get pregnant, anger toward pregnant women or women with babies, negative or self-deprecating comments concerning these feelings or other issues, isolation or avoidance of places where they might run into pregnant women or babies, and irritation. They may have difficulty concentrating and getting motivated at home or work.

It's also common for women to grieve after every menstrual cycle, and to feel a loss when their periods arrive. This grief process may take a very short time or can last longer. Recurrent periods of grief can lead to chronic grief or unresolved grief, and women and couples may feel that they are in limbo or out of control. The letdown associated with any new therapy that's unsuccessful can intensify the reaction.

Men are not necessarily better than women at handling issues of infertility. In addition to the grief they may feel, they often fear that they are letting their partners down.

"I often find that men are more concerned with taking care of their wives and don't allow themselves to concentrate on their own loss," says Pam Richey, M.S., a reproductive counselor and psychotherapist from Chapel Hill, North Carolina.

The Grief Process

Dealing with issues of infertility involves dealing with grief. Every person's experience of grief is different, so, obviously, there is no single cookie-cutter approach to working through it. There are, however, a few useful descriptions that seem to apply to many people who experience grief.

Probably the best-known analysis of the grieving process was introduced by Elisabeth Kübler-Ross in her book *On Death and Dying*, in which she identified the five stages of grief.[1] She interviewed people with terminal illnesses and found that most of them went through the following stages after learning that they were expected to die:

- Denial
- Anger
- Bargaining
- Depression
- Acceptance

These stages may be identified in many types of grief—not just grief related to death, but grief over any kind of loss. As regards infertility, grief may look something like this.

Denial

You feel numb. You don't think this could really be happening to you. There's no reason for you to be infertile! Your mom wasn't infertile. Your grandmother wasn't infertile. So obviously, there's been some sort of mistake here—right?

Anger

You may be angry with your partner ("Why did you smoke pot in college? I bet that's why we can't have a baby!"). You may be angry with your doctors for not solving your problem. You may be angry with God. You might also feel anger toward pregnant women, or toward your relatives with children. Every time you get a birth announcement, you may feel that it was sent with malice, to make you feel bad. Or every time you see a pregnant woman in a grocery store, you may think someone planted her there just to rub your face in your own troubles.

Bargaining

Bargaining is closely tied to guilt. Guilt is anger turned inward. You may be angry with yourself for past sexual experiences, past abortions, past activities, working too hard, not starting to try to conceive earlier—anything you think you might have done, even if it's ridiculously unlikely, that may be influencing your ability to get pregnant now. You may find yourself dwelling on regrets and fantasizing about going back in time to change your experiences. You may start wondering what terrible thing you've done to deserve this. You may feel guilty for "not trying hard enough."

This may be a time when you pray for a solution or fantasize about ways to solve the problem or "earn" your pregnancy. "I'll never drink again; I'll never yell at my husband again; I'll be a perfect mom and join the PTA," you might tell God or yourself. "Just let me have this and I'll never ask for anything again."

Depression

Like Eeyore's black rain cloud, depression hangs over everything in your life. You may feel that nothing will ever be okay again if you can't conceive children. The depression can be paralyzing, making even everyday activities feel like formidable chores. You may have trouble concentrating. You may have trouble with sleeping or eating—that is, you may sleep or eat too much or too little. You may feel irritable and oversensitive, or you may feel empty. Thoughts about infertility can consume you, making everything else seem pointless in comparison. This stage is probably the hardest; and it can be very difficult to pull out of depression and move on to the next stage, acceptance.

Acceptance

At this stage, you're able to put infertility into perspective. Most likely, you're not happy about it and are not willing to forget about it, but you can talk about it without breaking down. You can go on living and find worth in other areas of life. Maybe you are able to find joy in your favorite activities again, and you've stopped wanting to scream every time a coworker announces a pregnancy. Note that in this stage, you haven't necessarily stopped trying or stopped hoping; "acceptance" merely means that infertility doesn't rule your life anymore. This is why acceptance is often called the stage of "beginning again." You may find that your experience of loss can be very helpful to others facing similar losses. As you share your experiences with them, you may find that the contact is healing for you as well.

One criticism that some people make about these five stages, or any stages at all, is that grief rarely unfolds so neatly or so linearly. The stages are generalizations about what many people go through; but note that you may skip a stage, go through the stages backward, revert to an earlier stage after you've already passed through it once, or experience more than one stage at a time.

In other words, you may be depressed and angry at the same time, or feel guilt before you feel anger, or make it all the way through to acceptance only to have the process restart itself again when something triggers it, like a family member's pregnancy or your birthday or Mother's Day.

The stages are useful mostly as a way of recognizing that what you're going through is normal and a progressive process.

Other Reactions

Am I a Bad Person?

If you're feeling resentment toward pregnant women or secretly hoping that someone else won't conceive before you, this is normal.

It doesn't mean that you're a bad person. It means simply that you are grieving and wishing. Jealousy is to be expected. Sometimes it's hard not to feel as though you deserve a pregnancy more than someone else, so when you hear that your cousin who smokes and drinks and has been married for about 10 seconds got pregnant on her honeymoon, it's understandable that you may want to throw darts at her photo.

Logically, you know that someone else's pregnancy doesn't affect your own chances; your cousin hasn't used up part of this year's "baby quota." Acknowledge your feeling and do what you can to remind yourself that other people's pregnancies aren't meant to be a slap in your face.

"Wanting It Badly Enough"

For many successful women, this is the first time they haven't succeeded at something they've set their mind on. We're taught that if you want something badly enough and you work at it, you're supposed to be able to achieve it. Well, that works only in some areas—the ones you can control.

With fertility, some factors are under your control and some aren't. You may well do everything right and still not succeed, and that can be the most frustrating part of the situation. But you must believe that if you don't get pregnant, it's not because you didn't deserve a pregnancy.

Coping Mechanisms

The way you think and the beliefs you have about your infertility can help you cope or make it harder for you to cope. Here are a few tips:

- **Ease up on your expectations.** Sadness is often explained as unmet expectations. If, as each cycle begins, you expect to get pregnant this time, you're setting yourself up for disappointment. Any treatment you try may take more than a month to work. Of course you're going to feel hopeful each month, but try to remind yourself that you probably have many chances left if you don't get pregnant during this particular cycle.

- **Give up responsibility.** Take responsibility for the things you can control today, and let go of the rest. No matter how much you blame yourself for your past activities, you can't change history; and no matter how bad you feel about infertility that you didn't "cause," that feeling won't change your bodily functions. Feeling bad never helps anyone. If you don't blame yourself for having asthma, then don't blame yourself for infertility.

- **Examine your beliefs.** Some harmful beliefs come from our upbringing, our friends, our religion, or our own distortions of reality. What beliefs are hurting you? Do you believe that infertility makes you less of a woman or less of a wife? Do you believe that adoption is a less desirable option? Do you believe it's selfish to be childless, or that your life can't have meaning without children? None of these beliefs is true. Take time to think about which of these attitudes may be harming your self-esteem or mood, and work on cultivating healthier beliefs.

- **Grow closer.** Something good can actually come out of infertility. You may grow closer to your partner, friends, or family. You may find that someone who was just an acquaintance becomes a trusted friend. This won't happen if you withdraw, but it can happen if you open up and talk about your feelings. It's an honor for many people to feel trusted; when you talk about your private concerns with someone, that person may feel closer to you and privileged that you trusted him or her to advise or comfort you. And helping each other heal and cope with an imperfect situation creates stronger bonds within couples.

- **Think positively.** You can change your whole outlook on life by becoming aware of your negative thoughts and consciously replacing them with positive thoughts. If you find yourself thinking, "My life is worthless without a baby," write it down. Then cross it out and write down a positive thought to replace it. First, analyze the statement: Is it true? Has your life up until this point been worthless? Jot down the evidence that this statement is not true. What else provides meaning in your life? Have you helped anyone? Have you been a positive influence on anyone? What are you good at? What are your future goals? What else could you do to feel that your life means something?

- **Know your options.** There are many possible treatments for infertility. If one fails, that's not necessarily the end of the road. Research all your options, talk to couples who've gone through various treatments, and don't lose hope. Different things work for different people, and there's likely to be a solution for you.

- **Prepare yourself.** Regardless of how long you try and how many methods you use, there is a possibility that you won't have a successful pregnancy. Only you can decide how long you want to keep trying, how much money you want to spend on fertility treatments, and what degree of invasiveness you're willing to accept in a treatment. At some point, though, you'll need to weigh all this against your own emotional toll. If you and your partner are not depressed or overanxious, there's no problem. But if you find that it's taking too much out of you to get your hopes up every month and have them dashed, you may need to reconsider. Have a plan ready. Decide what you'll do if the situation gets to be too much. There are other ways to have children in your life— adopting, fostering, working at a day care center or school, becoming a mentor or "big sister," volunteering for child-related charities, etc. Or you may decide to remain child-free and fill your life with other things you love. Keep in mind that various possibilities exist, and that it won't be the end of your world if you cannot get pregnant.

Support Team

One of the best things you can do for yourself during this time is to put together a support team. This is a group of people who will be there for you as you work on this program and on any other fertility treatments.

Your Partner's Role

It's important to have a "fertility partner." Your spouse or life partner might be the preferable and most obvious choice for you, but sometimes issues of fertility can be hard for a partner to handle. Partners may be grappling with their own fertility issues and may find it difficult to hear the topic brought up. They may think they are expected to fix the problem, or that they are being blamed for it. And if your partner doesn't show as much emotion or talk about the situation as much as you do, resentment can build up in your relationship.

Also, your partner may be in a different stage of grief, or may have a different way of working through the issue. This doesn't mean that one of you cares more than the other, or is more affected by the problem. It just means that your coping mechanisms might work differently.

Effects of Infertility on Men

In the past, it was generally assumed that women find infertility more stressful than men do. However, researchers in Ireland weren't sure about this, so they gave 50 men in a fertility clinic a simple questionnaire to fill out. It measured levels of anxiety and depression.[2] They found that 31.9 percent of the men had detectable levels of anxiety, whether the fertility problem was male-factor, female-factor, or both. Clinically significant anxiety was found in 8.5 percent of the men, all of whom had a male-factor problem. None showed signs of clinical depression, however.

This result is important, because it raises a possibility many experts have come to believe—that it's more common for women to react to infertility with depression, and for men to react with anxiety.[3] If so, this may make it a little more difficult for a woman to notice that her male is affected; depression is more easily "seen," in crying, lethargy, lack of interest in activities and so on, whereas anxiety can be manifested in less obvious ways, such as dizziness, headaches, insomnia, and lack of patience or lack of concentration.

One stereotype, which seems to be true, is that men don't like to talk about their problems, letting things fester inside instead. A man may dearly want to be a father but may have trouble thinking about the obstacles and expressing his concerns.

Your Fertility Partner

That said, your fertility partner may be your significant other or a trusted friend or family member. Whoever it is must be willing and able to support you through diet, exercise, and any treatments that are necessary. This is your personal fertility cheerleader or fertility doula, so to speak. This person can be helpful in many ways.

- **Accountability.** Having someone to report to can keep you on track. Share your actions with this person; let him or her know how you're doing with your diet and exercise goals. Ask for encouragement when you need it. If you've written up an exercise schedule for the week, share it so that the person will know what you're aiming for. If the person wants to try the diet and exercise with you, great, but this isn't a condition of partnership.
- **Objective listening.** When people are deeply emotionally involved with an issue such as infertility, they often don't hear what physicians and counselors are telling them. If you're getting bad news, that may be all you hear—the bad news. An emotional

filter may be operating; and it's hard to concentrate on every detail you hear and every instruction you receive. Having a more objective partner attend appointments with you helps—he or she can take notes and later talk you through the information you may have missed during the appointment, or help you reframe the bits and pieces of advice you received. If you don't have this option, either bring a notebook and write down all the important points the doctor or counselor tells you, or ask if you can tape-record the conversation so that you can listen to it again later.

- **Hand-holding.** When you are dealing with difficult issues, it's nice just to have someone hold your hand and be there for you.

Your Doctor Works for You

If you're seeking help from a physician, remember that doctors are your consultants. They can offer recommendations, make predictions, and calculate the odds of success; but ultimately, the decisions about treatment are up to you. Many patients forget that doctors work for them, not the other way around. Your doctor is part of your fertility team, there to be consulted and to provide treatment. You have control over how you choose to proceed and which treatments you choose to pursue.

Women sometimes imagine that their doctor will fire them if they don't behave. What you should keep in mind instead is that you can fire your doctor if it's not a good match. It's important to have a good working relationship with your physician. You should be able to feel that you can ask questions about your treatment, and that the doctor is responsive, patient, and not dismissive of your concerns. He or she should feel comfortable discussing different treatment options with you.

Also, you might be reticent to ask about the clinic's rate of success because you're afraid of offending the doctor, but don't be. Simply ask, "Can you tell me your success rates with this procedure?"—but try not to get too hung up on the numbers. Often, an excellent clinic may have lower overall rates of pregnancy because it admits patients who are at higher risk of failure; some clinics will not treat women past a certain age, or women with poor prognoses. Some clinics favor more invasive and costly treatments with higher chances of success rather than trying simple treatments first.

You can get an objective overall picture of how your clinic compares to others, however. The Centers for Disease Control (CDC) now requires fertility clinics to report success rates, and you can find a statewide listing of these reports at www.cdc.gov/reproductive health/ART02/index.htm.

CDC warns consumers not to use the report to rank or grade fertility clinics, for exactly the reasons we just mentioned. CDC has advised: "For a more useful comparison, check for clinics that treated a higher percentage of couples similar to yours—those around the same age, with similar fertility problems, who used the same ART method you intend to use."[4]

One occasional problem is that a patient is afraid to tell the physician that she's not following the treatment program. Maybe she's having unwanted side effects or is finding the program too difficult. If this happens to you, don't be silent about it! Your doctor probably has other options for you, but he or she may not suggest them unless you are honest about your compliance or noncompliance with the treatments already suggested.

Again, remember that the doctor is not there to judge you, scold you, or force you into anything. You're in the driver's seat with regard to your treatment. If you don't feel that the doctor is on your team, or you don't feel comfortable discussing your concerns, it may be time to look for a different doctor.

Family

First, a note about parents. Your fertility may be a highly charged issue for your parents, and they may inadvertently put more pressure on you. Some parents can put their own wishes and expectations aside and fully be there for their kids; but often, parents won't be the best members of your core support team.

Siblings or other close relatives can often provide a tremendous amount of support. Just make sure that *they* are there for *you* on this issue, not vice versa. This is your time to be supported. If this is an emotionally charged issue for them, too, things can get complicated. You don't need any more complications. This is about you, not them.

People Say Stupid Things

Brace yourself. If you haven't already heard any stupid comments, you're likely to hear them at some point.

Nosy people who know you're trying to conceive may ask, "What's the problem? What's the holdup?"

Nosy people who don't know you're trying to conceive may ask when you're going to start trying, or why you haven't had kids (or more kids) yet, or make offhand and callous remarks about your "biological clock" and how you aren't getting any younger.

People who know you're having problems with fertility may ask why you're infertile, or spout advice about what their aunt did when she had these problems, or want to know why you don't "just adopt," or tell you how lucky you are that your life isn't burdened by diapers and that you can have one of their kids if you like.

What can we say? People are stupid.

No—most of these people are well intentioned; it's just that they don't understand. If they haven't been through infertility themselves, it can be hard for them to imagine what emotions you might be experiencing. Even if they have been through problems with fertility, your feelings and experiences may differ quite a bit from theirs.

How you handle such comments is entirely up to you. You may handle them with humor or sarcasm. You might simply say, "I don't want to discuss that" or "I'm sorry, but that's my personal business."

You might give a simple explanation that cuts the discussion short. You might say, "We're trying to have another child, and we'll let you know if it happens," or "I'm a little sensitive about that because we're trying to conceive."

Most people won't keep pressing the issue if you give some sort of answer, but if every time your coworker asks, "So? When are you two lovebirds going to have some kids?" you just smile and say, "I don't know," she may not have any idea that she's hurting you. She may think she's showing you that she cares; she may think that you appreciate it. You don't owe anyone any explanations or details, and of course you don't have to say a word; but for your own sake, the questions might quiet down if you simply say that it's a sensitive issue and you'd prefer not to talk about it.

Miscarriage

"I was told by my gynecologist that I had an extremely small chance of ever conceiving on my own, if at all, and that in order for me to ovulate and get pregnant I'd need to get on Clomid, and possibly metformin," says Lynette Peters. "I did not want to go the drug route, and at the time I was told this, decided to let things be. I started low-carbing to lose weight, never even knowing that it could and would help me get pregnant without the use of expensive, artificial drugs."

Lynette lost 42 pounds in three months and began ovulating normally for the first time in her life—and she got pregnant.

"Unfortunately, because I had low progesterone (a side effect of PCOS that I wasn't aware of until it was too late) I miscarried at six weeks," she says. "After the miscarriage, I got very depressed and my efforts fell by the wayside. It took me some time to get over it, and I don't think I'll ever completely be over it."

However, two years later, she decided to give it another try. She began a lifestyle that includes a low-carb diet, exercise, and writing a journal, and she began ovulating again. She's currently awaiting the results of a pregnancy test.

Grieving over a miscarriage is different for everyone, but it can be devastating. People who haven't been through this experience rarely know what to say or how to help. Find a therapist or a support group (in person or online) to help you through this pain. Only you will know if or when you're ready to try to conceive again.

Support Resources

There are many resources designed to offer support specifically for people dealing with issues of fertility.

ASRM

The American Society of Reproductive Medicine (ASRM) provides a directory of mental health professionals who specialize in reproductive failure. Visit the directory at www.asrm.org/search/providersearch.html to find a professional in your area. Seeing a therapist can help you learn to cope with your grief and can give you a safe place to let out any stress you might feel about infertility treatments, any anger you might feel toward insensitive people who've made stupid comments, or any other emotional issues you may be grappling with. If you lack a friend who's a "fertility partner," a therapist can also fill this role for you. You'll have someone to check in with to help keep you on track toward your diet and exercise goals.

Some therapists work only with individuals or couples; others also offer support groups. Fees vary widely, but some offer sliding-scale fees, and it's generally less expensive to join a group than it is to participate in individual or couples counseling. Make a few phone calls and see if you "click" with a therapist. Don't be afraid to change a therapist or a group if, after a couple of sessions, you don't think it's the right match.

Resolve

Resolve: National Infertility Association (www.resolve.org) is a nonprofit organization with a terrific number of resources. There are currently 50 chapters throughout the United States, most of which have their own websites listing local events and support groups.

Online membership is free and allows you to post on the message board, join online chats, and read the literature. The organization also offers consumer memberships for a fee, which includes access to a toll-free help line, medical call-in hours, local support groups and events, physician referrals, and a subscription to the quarterly magazine *Family Building*.

Online Groups

There are dozens of online groups for those who are trying to conceive or are dealing with infertility. Here's a sampling:

- www.fertilethoughts.com has several message boards and a chat room for women and men dealing with infertility.
- www.ttcdreams.com has an e-mail support group with more than 200 members.
- www.inciid.org/article.php?cat=forums&id=223 offers message boards on medical topics and general support topics.
- http://health.groups.yahoo.com/group/infertility-circle is an e-mail support group with nearly 300 members.

For low-carb support there are many websites where people exchange tips and recipes, offer general support for one another, and review products and share news related to the low-carb lifestyle. On lowcarbfriends.com, there's also an area for people who are trying to conceive (see "The Maintain Lane" section of the bulletin board), so you can find people who are in your exact situation.

Mind-Body Integration

There are many techniques you can try to reduce your stress and help bring joy back into your life.

Guided Imagery

Many tapes and CDs offer guided imagery. You may call them meditations, guided relaxation, or even hypnosis—they're all closely related concepts.

Typically, you'll hear slow, pretty instrumental music—piano, flute, guitar, maybe harp or bells—and a soothing male or female voice leading you through a "scene." The scene may be an idyllic nature setting, such as walking along a stream or standing atop a mountain; or it may be a theater, a house, or an abstract locale. Some recordings are meant to be heard through headphones only, whereas you can play others on any stereo equipment or even on your computer.

A guided relaxation session may last just a few minutes or up to an hour. Most tapes will advise you to sit or lie down, close your eyes, and consciously slow down and deepen your breathing. Some will advise you to tighten and flex your muscles in sequence to release tension.

One of our favorites is the Brain Sync series, which you can find at www.brainsync.com. We've used the "Spiritual Growth" tapes and found them very calming and easy to follow. You can sample a "Seven-Minute Brain Vacation" here: www.brainsync.com/relaxnow.asp.

Breathing Exercises

When we're stressed, we tend to take shallow breaths or even hyperventilate. This constricts our arteries, and we don't get enough oxygen to the brain or to the rest of the body. As a result, we find it hard to focus, and our anxiety is raised. For instant relief from stress, try some diaphragmatic breathing exercises.

To learn how to do this kind of exercise, lie on your back and put a book—maybe this one!—on your abdomen. When you inhale, try to raise the book. You want your breath to fill your belly, not just your chest. The goal is to fill your lungs from the lowest part to the highest part, not the reverse. Take in a slow, deep breath; hold it for three seconds; then exhale as slowly as you possibly can. The exhalation should be longer than the inhalation, like a long sigh.

You may want to add a word or phrase to your breathing exercises: For example, you might think "I can" when you inhale, and "let go" when you exhale, or just "relax" or "peace" when you exhale.

If you're not used to breathing this way, you may become light-headed the first few times you try. If that happens, just alternate—breathe normally for a minute, then take a few deep breaths again.

Once you get used to this exercise, you won't need a book and you won't even need to lie down; you'll be able to use this instant-relief technique while sitting or standing, no matter where you are.

Massage Therapy

Many people find that the best relaxation is hands-on! Find a certified massage therapist (check the yellow pages or ask around for recommendations) and pamper yourself with a massage. You might want a light-touch relaxation massage, or a deep-tissue Swedish massage. If you're uncomfortable about getting undressed, you don't have to. You can wear a T-shirt and shorts if you like; or you can get a seated (chair) massage, for which you can wear whatever you like (as long as it's not bulky).

You may also try Reiki, a very light hands-on form of healing and relaxation that's more spiritual in nature; its purpose is to heal your "life force energy" and many participants say that they feel as if light is radiating through them while they are undergoing a treatment. A

Reiki practitioner will probably lay hands on your head, abdomen, and feet.

Aromatherapy

Aromatherapy is the use of essential oils to alter moods or promote healing. Essential oils are distilled directly from the roots, leaves, bark, flowers, and stems of plants and are typically diluted with some kind of carrier oil (often almond oil) so as not to irritate the skin.

Several oils are recommended for relief of stress, the most common of which is lavender. You may also wish to try chamomile, ylang-ylang, sage, basil, jasmine, sandalwood, patchouli, and myrrh.

Aromatherapy products are available in many forms: lotions, bath beads, sprays, shampoos, and so on. Room diffusers are also available; these allow you to put a favorite oil or scented beads in a heated container or a device with a fan to disseminate the scent throughout a room.

You can also get creative. Try putting a few drops of your favorite oil on a tissue; then attach the tissue to your air-conditioning vent.

Just holding a vial of oil close to your nose can do the trick. Or you may want to add a few drops to boiling water, then turn off the heat and, keeping your face at least a foot away from the water, inhale the steam (with or without a towel over your head—the towel is helpful if you're trying to clear clogged sinuses).

Masseuses can also add essential oils to your massage treatment. Any oil you like can be added to neck wraps. If you have trouble relaxing before you go to sleep, try a lavender sleep mask or eye pillow.

If It Makes You Happy

Don't let problems with fertility become the focal point of your life. If you feel that those problems are getting dangerously close to taking over your life, step back and find something that brings you joy. Maybe there are hobbies you used to love—like skating, knitting, or painting—but haven't made time for in quite a while. Maybe there are things you've always wanted to try, like making ceramics or compiling a scrapbook or dancing, but you've never quite gotten around to. If you're a sports fan, get to some live games. If you like to sing, join a choir.

Doing good for others can also raise your mood and your sense of self-worth. Why not find a local charity and volunteer? Visit www .volunteermatch.org to find organizations in your area that are looking for volunteers. You might be surprised by the diversity of possibilities—everything from calling Bingo numbers at a senior center to weeding gardens, building homes, helping with secretarial work, and mentoring underprivileged children.

Take a vacation whenever you can, even if it's just a weekend away at a bed-and-breakfast in the next county. And keep yourself surrounded with friends, not just the ones who are there to offer a shoulder to cry on, but also the ones who make you laugh and not think too much.

Take time to do something you enjoy, something that brings you fulfillment, every day. This will help you remain centered.

Date Night

Last but not least, if you're going through this process with a partner, don't forget him or her. Even (and especially) during stressful times, it's important to take time to enjoy your spouse or partner. Nurture your relationship. Find things you both like to do and make time to do them. It doesn't have to cost a fortune to have a night out; it just has to be time for the two of you to leave some of the pressure behind and just hang out with each other. Remember, this relationship will be the foundation for the family you yearn to create. Let's keep that foundation healthy.

To this end, you may want to try some couples coaching or counseling.

"There can be conflict related to fertility, spoken and unspoken," says the reproductive counselor and psychotherapist Pam Richey. "A good marriage and family therapist versed in fertility issues can help couples strengthen their relationship and skills through adversity. This is great practice for how to relate with each other after the kids get here!"

Seven

Get Savvy About
Supplements
and Medications

i F YOU'VE EVER walked through the aisle of supplements at a pharmacy, you know that there are hundreds of pills, liquids, and tablets you can buy. They promise everything from clearer skin to the prevention of diseases, but which ones can do anything for your fertility, and which could actually harm you? Don't skip this—what you're about to read is crucial to this program and contains details of the latest research about what helps—and what to avoid.

Magnificent Minerals

Chromium

Chromium is one of 15 trace elements essential for proper metabolism of lipids and carbohydrates.

Chromium supplements lower glucose and insulin levels in normal, overweight, and diabetic individuals. I recommend 200 mcg. per day of organic chromium picolinate.

Researchers from Bastyr University in Washington State reported, "Serum glucose can be improved by chromium supplementation in both types 1 and 2 diabetes, and the effect appears dose dependent." They added, "The beneficial effects of chromium on serum glucose and lipids and insulin resistance occur even in the healthy."[1]

Chromium may also have beneficial effects on cholesterol and osteoporosis.

Magnesium

Magnesium doesn't have as clear a role as chromium in glucose metabolism; however, magnesium-rich diets and higher serum magnesium levels are associated with a lower risk of developing diabetes.

The researcher Mark McCarty was trying to figure out why whole grains are so much better for us than refined grains; whole-grain foods are known to reduce the risk of stroke, diabetes, and various types of cancer, among other health problems. Whole wheat flour also promotes insulin sensitivity, whereas white flour doesn't, yet their glycemic indexes are similar. To McCarty, this suggests that "certain nutrients or phytochemicals in whole wheat, depleted by the refining process, promote preservation of insulin sensitivity. Magnesium is a likely candidate in this regard."

Simply put, magnesium deficiency promotes insulin resistance, and supplementation improves insulin sensitivity.

Although it's not known just how magnesium works on insulin levels, it may act by antagonizing cellular calcium, which hinders the cellular signal of insulin if levels are too high.

You may take 250 mg. per day of supplemental magnesium. Whole-grain breads are also excellent sources of this mineral.

Amazing Amino Acids

L-Carnitine

L-carnitine is an amino acid that's important in mitochondrial transport of free fatty acids. Several studies have found that when L-carnitine is administered intravenously, it improves insulin-mediated glucose disposal,[2] free fatty acid disposal, and endothelial function in blood vessels.[3] (It's speculated that endothelial dysfunction plays a key role in developing insulin resistance because it limits how well insulin passes from the blood to the cells, where the effect is seen.)

Oral supplements of L-carnitine are available. ProXeed is marketed as a supplement for men with proven improvements in sperm count and motility. However, we were unable to find any data about the effects of oral L-carnitine supplements on insulin sensitivity.

L-carnitine is not recommended for people who take doxorubicin (Adriamycin, Rubex), isotretinoin (Accutane), valproic acid and derivatives (Depacon, Depakene, Depakote), or zidovudine (Retrovir).

N-Acetyl Cysteine

Two important studies of women with PCOS have found that N-acetyl cysteine has good effects. The first, a clinical study of 37 women in Italy, found that 1.8 grams per day of N-acetyl cysteine improved the insulin sensitivity of patients with PCOS.[4]

The second study, completed in 2005, involved 150 infertile women with PCOS who had not responded to clomiphene citrate (brand names: Clomid, Serophene), a drug used to stimulate ovulation. The researchers added 1.2 grams of N-acetyl cysteine per day to the women's treatment and found that it significantly increased both ovulation rate and pregnancy rate: 49.3 percent ovulated (versus 1.3 percent in the placebo group), and 21.3 percent achieved pregnancy (versus 0 percent in the placebo group).[5] They reported that the supplement was safe and well tolerated, and that it did not cause ovarian hyperstimulation syndrome when used in conjunction with clomiphene citrate.

Worth trying? Absolutely.

Essential Fatty Acids

Alpha-Lipoic Acid

Alpha-lipoic (ALA) is crucial in our mitochondria, too. It protects the mitochondria and our DNA, and when there's "leftover" ALA (there usually isn't, unless we get it in supplement form), it acts as an antioxidant.

Numerous studies have found that both intravenous supplementation and oral supplementation of ALA improve glucose disposal and insulin sensitivity.[6] You can take an oral dose of up to 600 mg. per day—there's no benefit to taking a higher dose.

Mitochondrial Factor

Coenzyme Q10

This antioxidant increases mitochondrial functioning. It's being studied as a treatment or preventive measure for type 2 diabetes, with suggestions that it's more effective when started earlier in the disease.[7]

Studies have indicated that it improves insulin sensitivity.[8] There are no direct data on its impact on women's fertility; there is some research suggesting a positive impact on sperm function in subfertile men.[9]

Heavenly Herbals

Chaste Tree

Extracts from chaste tree berries (*Vitex agnus-castus*) have been shown to have several hormonal properties, including antiestrogen activity similar to the fertility medicine clomiphene citrate (brand names: Clomid, Serophene).

Two placebo-controlled studies found a modest improvement in pregnancy rates, as well as improvements in progesterone production and menstrual cyclicity.

A word of caution: One report found that the extracts had some antiprogesterone activity. This could potentially lead to poor implantation and miscarriage once pregnancy is achieved. We recommend taking this preparation for only the first 14 days of the menstrual cycle, then stopping it.

Also, if you're taking Clomid, *don't* take chaste tree berry; they work in a similar fashion and could result in ovarian hyperstimulation.

Ginger

One experiment has found that ginger can improve insulin sensitivity.[10] A second clinical trial found no improvement in blood lipids or blood sugar when patients with coronary artery disease took 4 grams daily for three months. This is one of those supplements that might help and can't hurt. Ginger also has a proven ability to combat the nausea that often occurs with pregnancy. You can use fresh ginger in foods or tea, or take it in supplemental form.

Ginseng

Similarly, ginseng has shown some beneficial properties as regards insulin. A clinical study of 36 non-insulin-dependent diabetic patients in 1995 concluded, "Ginseng therapy elevated mood, improved psychophysical performance, and reduced fasting blood glucose (FBG) and body weight." Patients took either 100 or 200 mg. daily for eight weeks.[11]

Although many studies of ginseng were animal studies (whose results can't always be generalized to humans), several trials found that ginseng improved insulin sensitivity.[12] Another trial found that ginseng was only "marginally active" in improving insulin function.[13] *Ginseng is generally well tolerated, but it has a few contraindications, so be sure to consult with your doctor before you begin supplementing your diet with ginseng.*

Royal Jelly

Royal jelly is a nutrient-rich compound said to have many beneficial features, mostly related to lowering cholesterol and improving the immune system. It's the food of bee royalty: the queen bee's favorite dish, and the substance that turns an ordinary bee into a queen bee. The worker bees secrete this milky substance—which is a mix of glandular chemicals, digested pollen, and honey or nectar—and place it in the queen cells of the hive for the nourishment of the developing larval queen bee. It's full of vitamin B.

The worker bees get royal jelly only for the first few days of their lives; thereafter, they just get pollen and honey. The point of royal jelly is to make the queen bee extra-fertile: while the workers feed her, she may lay up to 2,000 eggs each day. One study done on ewes found that royal jelly supplementation improved ovulation and pregnancy rates.[14] It may sound strange, but of all mammals, ewes have the placental physiology closest to that of humans. So although this is not human evidence, it's a good sign.

All bee products may cause allergic reactions (such as asthma attacks and skin irritations), so royal jelly is not recommended if you are allergic to pollen, bee stings, or honey. It's also not recommended for pregnant or

lactating women. No recommended dosage levels have been estab-
lished, but most manufacturers suggest 500 mg. twice a day.

Other Herbs

There are many other herbs with possible benefits for women's
health and fertility; these include traditional Chinese medicine
(TCM). However, no well-designed studies to evaluate their effectiveness can be found in the medical literature. This, of course, does
not mean that there may not be benefit from some of these agents,
but it also means that there may be untoward effects that haven't
been discovered. At present, there are none of these other agents
that we would recommend, and we would suggest that you refrain
from using them until a more detailed assessment of risks and benefits of particular agents is available.

Tea for Two—as Long as It's Green

Since we've told you that you need to cut down on coffee, why not
switch to tea? New studies have found that green and oolong teas
actually help fight insulin resistance, with green tea having the
greatest impact.

Green tea has long been credited with anticarcinogenic, antioxidant, and anti-inflammatory properties, but now it's also said to be
an antidiabetic agent and a fertility booster.

Green tea does contain caffeine, which is known to decrease insulin sensitivity, but that effect seems to be overruled by a chemical
called epigallocatechin gallate.

In Japan and China, researchers found that green tea substan-
tially improved people's glucose tolerance.[15] Scientists at the U.S.
Department of Agriculture (USDA) have said that green tea improves insulin activity more than 15-fold.[16] The results were the
same whether the tea contained caffeine or was decaffeinated.

Research on black tea has had mixed results. This is fully fermented green tea, and in the fermentation process the tea seems to lose its insulin-sensitizing effects. The impact on insulin is also negated when you drink your tea with dairy, soy milk, or nondairy creamer. Lemon juice is fine to add, though.

Hold the Herbal Teas

Herbal teas are not actually from the tea plant, so technically they are just brews. Depending on the herbs, herbal brews may or may not affect insulin sensitivity. Because herbal ingredients aren't subject to approval by the FDA, few of them have undergone clinical testing to determine what their positive and negative effects might be.

Dietary Fertility Boosters

Fiber

Several recent epidemiologic studies have found that people with higher-fiber diets have less insulin resistance.[17]

In 2003, researchers at the University of South Carolina interviewed 978 adults about their food habits and found that the more whole grain (dark breads, high-fiber and cooked cereals) they ate, the better their insulin sensitivity was.[18]

Fiber slows the absorption of sugars from the gut, preventing a large insulin surge after your meal (reactor rods work similarly in a nuclear power plant to slow the nuclear reaction).

Your fiber intake is easy to track by reading "Nutritional Facts" labels, and you should aim for at least 20 grams per day.

Buckwheat

Buckwheat seeds are rich in the compound D-chiro-inositol (dCI), and dCI makes up as much as 40 percent of the carbohydrate content of buckwheat flour.[19]

DCI supplementation (600 mg. per day) in women with PCOS resulted in a 33 percent drop in insulin levels, a 73 percent drop in testosterone, and an ovulation rate three times higher, compared with women taking a placebo.[20] So, particularly if you have PCOS, stock up on buckwheat! And even if you don't have PCOS, dietary buckwheat or dCI supplements will be likely to improve your fertility.

Spice It Up!

Cinnamon

Call it a happy accident. Richard Anderson and his team at the USDA's Human Nutrition Research Center were investigating the effects of common foods on blood sugar levels. One of the foods they tested was apple pie. Of course, they expected blood sugar to skyrocket after such a sweet dessert—but it had the opposite effect. It actually improved insulin action.[21]

This was quite a surprise, but the team finally figured out that the cinnamon in the apple pie was causing the positive effects. Cinnamon contains the compound methylhydroxy chalcone polymer (MHCP), which makes fat cells more responsive to insulin.

Some of the same researchers conducted a study in Pakistan in 2003 to find out just how effective cinnamon could be for people with type 2 diabetes. They gave 30 people either 1, 3, or 6 grams of cinnamon in capsule form for 40 days. Another 30 people received a placebo. What did the researchers discover? Just half a teaspoon of cinnamon a day significantly reduced blood sugar, triglyceride, LDL cholesterol, and total cholesterol.

They also discovered that cinnamon oil doesn't have the desired effect on insulin, but cinnamon powder and cinnamon sticks both work. One of the researchers, a nondiabetic, found that his own blood sugar levels went down after he drank tea flavored with a cinnamon stick.

Cinnamon has a host of other known health benefits, including antibacterial properties and improvement of digestion.

If you don't like the taste of cinnamon, you can buy empty gelatin capsules, fill them with cinnamon powder, and swallow them as you would any supplement. If you do like the taste of cinnamon, start sprinkling it on everything from oatmeal to chicken. (No, this isn't a good excuse to run out for a cinnamon bun and a stack of French toast!)

For some helpful recipes that include cinnamon, visit http://answers.google.com/answers/threadview?id=308715.

Other Spices

Though none have proved to be as effective as cinnamon, there are other spices that have been found to improve insulin action in clinical studies. Among them are allspice, nutmeg, cloves, and turmeric.

These spices tend to be rich in chromium, although the proportion of chromium didn't necessarily correlate with which spices performed best. Cinnamon contained the highest amount of chromium: 1,818 nanograms per gram.[22]

Complementary Therapy: Acupuncture

Acupuncture is based on ancient Asian medical theory; however, recent research has unraveled some of its therapeutic secrets, and it may have a beneficial role in fertility.

In women, acupuncture leads to changes in endogenous opioid production in the brain that can in turn lead to improvements in the hormonal control of ovulation.[23] One study of 24 women with PCOS and oligoamenorrhea found that 10 to 14 electro-acupuncture treatments induced regular ovulation in more than one-third of the women. The women who had good results from this treatment had a significantly lower BMI and a better hormonal profile than they had before the study began.[24]

Another study, at Shanghai Medical Institute in China, concluded, "Clinical observation showed that electro-acupuncture with the effective acupoints could cure some anovulatory patients [at] a highly effective rate."[25]

Acupuncture has also been found to decrease vascular resistance in the uterus of infertile women to improve uterine blood flow, which may improve implantation.[26]

Also of interest is that in a controlled clinical trial, acupuncture has been found to improve sperm motility in subfertile men.[27] In a separate study, researchers measured sperm concentration, volume, and motility before and after men's acupuncture treatments, and found a significant increase in sperm quality in all measurements but volume.[28]

In short, many researchers studying acupuncture have examined surrogate markers for potential fertility and have suggested a favorable effect. There is little evidence to date, however, that definitively shows improved chances of taking home a baby. Until such data are obtained, we can say only that acupuncture appears to be of benefit and has few drawbacks, but how much benefit it may offer, if any, is unclear.

What to Avoid

Conjugated Linoleic Acid (CLA)

Conjugated linoleic acid (CLA) has been found to have benefits for weight loss and heart disease, and it is therefore a common ingredient in weight-loss supplements. However, there are different isomers of CLA, and they've had different effects. Several new clinical studies have found that CLA supplements hinder insulin metabolism and worsen insulin resistance in humans.

As we are mostly interested in improving insulin metabolism to improve the prospects of fertility, it would be prudent not to take CLA as an additional supplement.

Vitamin E

Don't gasp. We're not suggesting that you avoid anything that contains vitamin E. It's a great antioxidant, but its effects on insulin activity are a little uncertain. Some reports indicate improved insulin function with vitamin E, but some actually indicate worse function. Further, there are some reports in the oncology literature that indicate benefits for cancer patients because vitamin E has hindered cell division. This is not good as far as reproduction is concerned. So although you should get your recommended dietary allowance of vitamin E (15 mg. a day for women and men[29]), don't load up on it by specifically adding a vitamin E supplement to your regimen.

Smoking

Nearly everyone acknowledges that cigarette smoking leads to lung and heart disease, but most people don't realize that it also has specific affects on women's reproductive functions. To test public knowledge, researchers at Yale University School of Medicine surveyed 388 people who were in a position to know better: female hospital employees.

What the researchers discovered was that only 22 percent of the women realized that smoking has a negative impact on fertility and miscarriage, and only 25 percent realized that it increases the risk of ectopic pregnancy.[30]

Smoking is said to be responsible for approximately 13 percent of infertility,[31] 16 percent of miscarriages,[32] and a 3.5-fold increase in the risk of ectopic pregnancy.[33]

As if that's not bad enough, smoking increases the rate of egg depletion, thus also leading to earlier onset of menopause; it increases genetic damage to eggs and resultant embryos; and it decreases tubal motility.

There's also a noted link between smoking and insulin resistance. More than a decade ago, researchers in the United Kingdom discovered that chronic cigarette smokers are significantly more insulin-resistant than nonsmokers.[34]

Given all this, we hereby issue a strong recommendation for all couples with fertility failure to quit smoking by any means necessary as soon as possible. Quitting will improve your chance of becoming fertile, increase your capability for exercise, increase your likelihood of a healthy pregnancy, and improve your general health. You may put off quitting until you conceive, but it will probably be no fun to go through nicotine withdrawal at the same time as you go through morning sickness. Get it over with now—you won't regret it.

SMOKING CESSATION PROGRAMS

Many state and town governments sponsor smoking cessation support groups. Ask your doctor if he can recommend a local program.

Nicotine Anonymous borrows the 12-step program from Alcoholics Anonymous, and has more than 500 local chapters throughout the United States and online at www.nicotine-anonymous.org. Check there to see if there's a group near you. There are even some phone meetings available.

QuitNet at www.quitnet.com has online forums, a chat room, a service for finding a "quit buddy," a way to record your quit date anniversary, and more. The basic membership is free; a premium membership, which does involve a fee, includes advice from professional counselors along with a few extra features.

The American Lung Association's Freedom from Smoking cessation program is also available free online at www.lungusa.org.

NICOTINE REPLACEMENT PRODUCTS

Patches, gum, inhalers, and sprays—which should you choose?

Honestly, whichever you like.

In 1999, 504 volunteers at a hospital smoking clinic were randomly chosen to try either nicotine gum, transdermal patches, nasal spray, or inhalers for 12 weeks. Between 20 and 24 percent of those on the program were able to quit for those 12 weeks, regardless of the method used. The researchers concluded, "There are no notable differences between the products in their effects on withdrawal discomfort, perceived helpfulness, or general efficacy."[35]

Many people ask me if these products are safe. Well, they're a lot safer than smoking. Safety depends on how you use them, as well. For example, if you go on the patch and continue smoking anyway, that's not safe—you're overloading your body with nicotine. But if you use the products as intended, they deliver a low level of nicotine to keep your craving down without filling your body with the several thousand other chemicals present in cigarettes.

BUPROPION

Zyban and Wellbutrin are two commercial names of the prescription drug bupropion hydrochloride. They were both originally intended to treat depression, and they fall into the antidepressant class of medications. However, they have been found to significantly improve physical withdrawal symptoms for those who want to quit smoking. This effect was discovered by accident when people who were taking the medication for depression reported that they had much less desire for cigarettes. The medications contain no nicotine, and numerous clinical studies have found that they help twice as many smokers quit as placebos.[36] You can go on one of these medications in addition to using a nicotine replacement product; some studies have found a slightly higher success rate when these two methods are combined.[37]

You'll need a prescription, so talk to your doctor to see if either of these medications is appropriate for you.

Douching

A study of 840 women found that in comparison with nondouchers, women who douched were 30 percent less likely to become pregnant each month they attempted pregnancy.[38] It didn't matter what type of douche preparation they used, and douching affected young women's pregnancy rates more than those of older women (there was a 50 percent reduction for women 18 to 24 years old, a 29 percent reduction for women 25 to 29 years old, and a 6 percent reduction for women 30 to 39 years old).

Douching may also increase the risk of pelvic inflammatory disease, and one study of 611 women reported that the risk of tubal ectopic pregnancy for women who douched at least weekly was twice that of women who never douched.[39]

Douching may create a hostile environment in which it is difficult for sperm to survive. It's best avoided while you are trying to conceive, particularly around the time of ovulation.

Retinoids

If you're taking any oral retinoids, stop!

Accutane, prescribed for acne, and Soriatane, prescribed for psoriasis, have both been linked to severe risks of birth defects—so much so that the manufacturer goes to great lengths to ensure that doctors won't prescribe the medications for women unless the women have had a pregnancy test first. The generic versions carry the same recommendations. Soriatane remains in the system long after treatment has ended, so *women should not take this medication if they're thinking about conceiving within three years.*

According to the March of Dimes, all oral retinoids entail a risk of birth defects and should never be used by pregnant women. Although topical retinoids (like Retin-A) are less risky, the March of Dimes suggests that women avoid even these, as there is a possibility that the medication could get into the bloodstream. It suggests that women use, instead, topical preparations of the antibiotics erythromycin, clindamycin, or benzoyl peroxide as a first choice; and if the skin doesn't clear up, a doctor can prescribe oral antibiotics as a second choice.

Remember: Just because you can get supplements without a prescription, it doesn't mean they're free of side effects that could harm fertility. And on the flip side, just because a manufacturer claims a supplement will increase your fertility, it doesn't mean it's ever been proven. When in doubt, ask your doctor about supplements you're considering using to boost your fertility. Some supplements can help, others can just drain your bank account . . . or worse—harm your chances of a successful pregnancy.

Eight

Testing and Conventional Treatments

*i*N THE UNITED States, an estimated nine million couples (18 million people) are evaluated for infertility each year. Research polls find that there are many other couples who have not sought a formal evaluation for their infertility or who are not aware that they're infertile.

According to the American Fertility Association, about two-thirds of all couples who seek treatment will eventually have a child.

How It Happens

There are certain things Mom and Dad don't tell you when they sweat through "the talk." Sure, you know the basic concept of how to get pregnant, but did you know how much is going on in your body every day in preparation for this great feat?

A typical menstrual cycle is 21 to 35 days and is biphasic: that is, it goes through two stages. We'll use a 28-day cycle as our model, but the times may be adjusted if your cycle is shorter or longer. The two phases—before and after ovulation—are timed about evenly, at approximately 14 days per phase.

The Follicular Phase

The first day of your cycle is the day your period starts. The blood comes from the lining of the uterus, the endometrium, which is shedding itself because pregnancy has not occurred on the last cycle. The endometrium had thickened to prepare for implantation, but now it's ready to start again. Gonadotropin-releasing hormone (GnRH) produced in the hypothalamus—a part of the brain— signals the release of follicle-stimulating hormone (FSH), which is produced by the pituitary gland and tells the ovaries to grow follicles. The eggs are located in these follicles. Although several follicles (possibly 10 to 20) will typically grow, one will become dominant and the rest will recede.

Estrogen is low during the first part of the cycle. As you get closer to ovulation, follicles release estrogen to help the endometrium begin to thicken again to create a more welcoming environment for implantation to take place.

Ovulation

Ovulation is the most fertile time of the cycle. Luteinizing hormone from the pituitary gland signals the dominant follicle to rupture and release its egg (ovum), which travels through one of the fallopian tubes. The follicle then becomes the corpus luteum. The cervix feels soft and high during this time, and the opening widens. The cervical mucus is abundant, thin, and stretchy, often described as similar to raw egg whites.

During ovulation, some women experience mittelschmerz (mid-pain), which is mild pain or cramping in the abdomen, sometimes just on one side. There may also be spotting (light bleeding) around this time.

Progesterone causes the body temperature to rise slightly for the remainder of the cycle. The egg lives for only 12 to 24 hours if it doesn't get fertilized; then it disintegrates. Although this is a small window of opportunity, sperm can live up to five days in optimal conditions, so intercourse doesn't necessarily need to take place during ovulation for conception to happen.

The Luteal Phase

Progesterone causes the endometrium to change, preparing to support an embryo during the first few days of this phase. It also prevents the ovary from releasing another egg during the same cycle. If implantation doesn't happen, estrogen and progesterone levels drop, and the endometrium begins breaking down again.

If implantation does happen, the embryo releases human chorionic gonadotropin (hCG), which sustains the corpus luteum. The corpus luteum continues to produce progesterone to support the pregnancy.

Female-Factor Infertility

The two main physical causes of female infertility are ovulatory dysfunction and anatomic abnormalities.

Ovulatory Dysfunction

First, a lack of ovulation is obviously a problem. If you're having a regular period, and if you have all the typical symptoms that come along with menstruation (like cramps and premenstrual mood swings), the chances are good that you are ovulating. Still, this doesn't mean that you're ovulating *well*.

One of my patients, Beth Adams, suspected that something was wrong despite the fact that she had monthly periods.

"I always had a feeling that there was something not quite right because I've never had a cramp any day in my life. I never had PMS or anything like that, and all my friends did," she says.

That's not usually something a woman would complain about—until she's searching for reasons for her infertility. Although Beth had seemingly normal monthly periods, she was not ovulating. A review of her cycles showed that urine LH tests (ovulation predictor kits) had turned positive only sporadically. Upon doing an ultrasound and finding cysts all over her ovaries, I diagnosed PCOS. After treatment, Beth and her husband are now expecting their first baby.

If your cycles have become longer or shorter or you're missing periods, you may have ovulatory problems.

Ovulatory dysfunction may be caused by PCOS, the most common hormonal problem in women of reproductive age. This is characterized by a lack of ovulation combined with excess testosterone, and women with PCOS often (but not always) have excess hair growth, weight problems, and insulin resistance.

Thyroid disease can also cause ovulatory problems. Usually it's low thyroid function that causes trouble with reproduction, but high thyroid function can also cause problems.

Another culprit is high prolactin levels. Prolactin is a hormone with several functions, but its main purpose is to stimulate development of the mammary glands and induce milk production after pregnancy. The level of prolactin is supposed to go up during and after pregnancy, but stay fairly low otherwise. Excessive prolactin can cause amennorhea and other menstrual disruptions, and may be associated with hypothyroidism, kidney disease, and several other medical conditions.

There's also the possibility of declining ovarian function that's either age-related or premature. As eggs age, they become more prone to defects that can cause problems both with fertility and with fetal development.

A woman is born with about 500,000 immature eggs. Of these, about 300 will be released. For every egg that is released, about 1,000 others were "on call" and began maturing, but weren't deemed the "lucky" egg that was the strongest and most mature for its cycle.

The rest of the eggs undergo cell death or atresia, which is a degeneration that makes the eggs unusable. When a woman begins menopause, although she may have a few hundred eggs left, it's unlikely that those eggs will mature and be released.

Smoking can accelerate atresia. Early menopause may be caused by cancer treatments, autoimmune disorder (in which the body builds up antibodies and begins mistakenly attacking its own organs or cells), or chromosomal abnormalities, or it may be unexplainable.

Anatomical Abnormalities

Several anatomical abnormalities may cause or contribute to infertility.

Prior infections, surgeries, or endometriosis may lead to tubal obstruction. Endometriosis is a condition in which the tissue that normally lines the uterus implants itself outside the uterus in the pelvis or abdominal area. It often, though not always, causes painful menses or painful intercourse, and it can lead to inflammation and scarring that hinder fertility.

Most commonly, pelvic infections (which are often undetected) cause tubal damage in the form of blockages or bands of scar tissue. These infections may be a result of past childbirth, miscarriage, STDs, or even tuberculosis.

Likewise, several problems can lead to uterine abnormalities. Within the uterine cavity, there may be submucus fibroids, which most women who have them don't know they have because they don't have symptoms. Fibroids are benign (noncancerous) tumors that can be pea-size or can grow much larger, and are most common in women in their thirties and forties and in overweight women.

Most fibroids don't interfere with fertility or pregnancy; their effect depends on their size and location. If the fibroid develops on the wall or outside surface of the uterus (as most fibroids do), it's not a problem. Fibroids become a problem only when they are inside the uterine cavity and are large, sometimes blocking or pressing on reproductive passages. If symptoms are present, they may include heavy menstrual bleeding, anemia, painful intercourse, pressure in the abdomen, lower back pain, and bladder problems.

Intrauterine adhesions, or scar tissue in the uterus, can interfere with implantation of an embryo and can also cause miscarriage. Such adhesions can be caused by infection after abortion or after gynecological surgery.

Uterine polyps—extra pieces of tissue in the uterine lining that are somewhat like skin tags—can interfere with fertility if they are large or abundant. They tend to grow when estrogen levels are high.

A uterine septum is a malformation of the uterus. In this condition a dividing wall extends down part or all of the inside of the uterus and can interfere with fertility and pregnancy. The larger the septum, the more likely it is to cause trouble.

If you have structural damage that requires surgical intervention, chances are that no amount of proper diet and exercise will fix it, though the program in this book can certainly help restore your fertility once any obstructions are removed.

Then there are the 33 percent or so of couples who have "unexplained infertility"—that is, all of the tests are normal for both partners.

Basic Fertility Tests

Testing is meant to check for common causes of infertility like those we just mentioned. Both partners should undergo testing. (Remember that infertility is just as likely to be a male-factor problem as a female-factor problem).

Tests for Women

Testing for women may include the following:

- *Medical history.* You and your partner will be interviewed or will fill out a questionnaire about any prior illnesses or surgeries, current medical conditions, medications you're taking (remember to include herbal supplements and over-the-counter medications, even if the doctor doesn't ask about these), sexual history, past pregnancies, and so on.
- *A physical exam.* This is a whole-body general physical, including a gynecological exam.
- *Basal body temperature (BBT) or urinary ovulation predictor kits.* A BBT test is a chart of a woman's waking temperature to determine when ovulation occurs. A urinary stick test can also determine the timing of ovulation.
- *Selected laboratory blood tests.* Depending on the clinical scenario, there are many simple blood tests that may be done. Doctors can check your thyroid function and your levels of various hormones (prolactin, estrogen, testosterone, luteinizing, progesterone, etc.) just by taking a blood sample from your arm. Many of these tests need to be timed according to parts of your menstrual cycle. Your doctor may also order a clomiphene challenge test, which is a test of the quality of eggs left in your ovaries. Androgen testing, which checks levels of free and total testosterone and dihydroepiandrosterone sulfate (DHEAS), may be used to help diagnose PCOS,

hypothalamic dysfunction, or pituitary gland dysfunction. Insulin and glucose tests may also be done; however, many doctors don't regularly screen for insulin resistance, because it's difficult to measure.

- *Ultrasound.* This noninvasive test is used to check for fibroids in the uterus and for follicle growth or the presence of cysts in the ovaries. It is also used to examine the thickness of the uterine lining (this affects implantation).
- *HSG X Ray.* This X ray, called a hysterosalpingogram, inspects the fallopian tubes and uterus to check for blockages and structural abnormalities. A dye is injected through the cervix to highlight any problems. If the dye doesn't pass through both ends of the fallopian tubes, there's probably a blockage. This test may cause mild discomfort or pain. (Be sure to take 800 mg. of ibuprofen beforehand to minimize the cramps—that is, as long as you don't have a problem with ibuprofen, in which case your doctor can give you something else.)
- *Laparoscopy.* In specific clinical situations, a doctor may perform a laparoscopy, an outpatient procedure in which a thin scope is inserted in a woman's abdomen so that the doctor can look at the reproductive organs to check for scarring or endometriosis.

Tests for Men

In addition to the medical history and physical exam, tests for men may include these.

- *Semen analysis.* The man ejaculates into a container, and the semen is studied for sperm count, volume, motility, forward progression, acidity, and shape, as well as potential infections.
- *Hormonal blood tests.* Abnormal hormone levels can interfere with sperm production.
- *Anti-sperm antibody tests.* These tests can determine whether the woman is producing antibodies to attack the man's sperm, or

whether the man is producing antibodies that attack his own sperm.

- *Testicular biopsy.* The doctor will take a small tissue sample from the testicles and inspect it to check sperm production.
- *Sperm DNA fragmentization test.* This is a new test that is being looked at by researchers. It is intended to measure the percentage of sperm cells in which the DNA has been broken up. Early studies have found a strong correlation between this condition and the inability to achieve a successful pregnancy; however, the issue is still being investigated. This test may give insight into particularly perplexing cases.
- *Chromosomal testing.* Certain genetic disorders are associated with severely low sperm counts. Microdeletions in certain regions of the Y chromosome can lead to low counts and even to a complete absence of sperm. Other problems, such as Klinefelter's syndrome (in which there are two X chromosomes and one Y chromosome), and a condition in which the Y chromosome is shaped like a ring, can also lead to low counts. Generally, if a man's sperm count is consistently less than 5 million sperm per milliliter, he should be offered genetic testing.

Common Fertility Treatments

Regardless of the cause, treatment revolves around having a good-quality egg to fertilize and sperm that are capable of doing the job.

Induction of Ovulation

A number of medicines may induce ovulation. The most common are clomiphene citrate (Clomid and Serophene) and, recently, letrozole (Femara). They work similarly, but clomiphene is less expensive and has a longer track record for effectiveness. There has long been concern that Clomid has a negative effect on the uterine lining, and it is true that the average lining is slightly thinner compared with its condition in a natural cycle. Its thickness, however, is still in the normal range—and women who have been infertile do get pregnant more often when they take this medicine. There are a few individuals for whom this issue is more prominent, and they may require a different form of therapy.

Either Clomid or Femara is prescribed for five days toward the beginning of each menstrual cycle. Both medicines are associated with mild side effects (such as hot flashes, blurred vision, mood swings, headache, and nausea) and rare complications (multiple births, ovarian cysts).

If the pills don't work, your doctor may prescribe injections of follicle-stimulating hormone (FSH), to encourage the growth of follicles that will help eggs mature. Although these injections achieve higher pregnancy rates than the pills, they are also more likely to have adverse effects, such as multiple births, ovarian hyperstimulation syndrome (in which women can develop fluid shifts and electrolyte abnormalities), or large ovarian cysts.

The chance of a pregnancy in a given month after a year of unsuccessful attempts is roughly 1 to 2 percent. Treatment with Clomid raises the chance to 5 to 8 percent. Gonadotropins raise it to 12 to 15 percent. Multiple births (twins, triplets, etc.) occur in 8 percent to 17 percent of births resulting from the use of fertility drugs—8 percent in the case of Clomid, 17 percent in the case of gonadotropins.[1]

Artificial Insemination (AI)

Artificial insemination is the process of placing "washed" sperm (the healthiest, strongest, fastest sperm that have been processed from a man's semen) directly into the uterine cavity while the woman is ovulating. This way, the sperm bypasses the vagina and cervix (and potentially hostile cervical mucus). Under normal circumstances, roughly 500 to 1,000 sperm will reach the fallopian tubes, where the egg awaits fertilization. AI places millions of sperm in the upper genital tract to enhance the chance that one lucky sperm will find the single egg.

AI is a relatively simple procedure, similar to a Pap smear, that shouldn't cause much discomfort. It may be done with or without the help of ovulation-stimulating medicines.

This technique significantly raises the chances of pregnancy when there is mild male-factor infertility or unexplained infertility. It brings the chance with Clomid up to 8 to 12 percent and the chance with gonadotropins up to 18 to 20 percent.

Typically, this process uses the husband's sperm, but donor sperm may be used if the husband's semen contains few or no moving sperm.

In Vitro Fertilization (IVF)

There are five steps in IVF.

First, the woman injects herself with hormones to stimulate the ovaries, in the hope that they'll produce more than one egg. She also takes medication to make sure that the eggs are not actually released before the doctor retrieves them. During this time, she's closely monitored to make sure that hyperstimulation of the ovaries doesn't occur (ovarian hyperstimulation syndrome can be very dangerous). Just before the eggs are to be retrieved, she takes human chorionic gonadotropin (hCG), a medication that stimulates the final maturation of the follicles.

Second, about two hours before the eggs are retrieved, the man provides a semen sample, and the sperm are washed.

Third, the eggs are retrieved. Typically, doctors accomplish this step by inserting a vaginal probe and removing the eggs through a needle. Sometimes retrieval requires a laparoscopy under general anesthesia.

Fourth, any eggs that are healthy are placed in a lab dish with the sperm, in the hope that some eggs will be fertilized. If they are, the embryos are cultured for several days in the lab.

Fifth, the embryos are inserted directly into the woman's uterus through a catheter, bypassing the fallopian tubes. Generally, two to four embryos are used. Any leftover embryos may be frozen for future use so that the entire procedure will not need to be repeated if the initial attempt fails. Most embryos will survive the freezing and thawing process.

One type of IVF is intracytoplasmic sperm injection (ICSI), in which one sperm is injected directly into an egg to create an embryo. This is done when a severe male factor is present. ICSI brings the chance of successful fertilization up to normal, thus giving couples with male-factor infertility an excellent chance at a pregnancy. A common question that arises is whether ICSI selects out defective sperm that could lead to a higher risk of birth defects. However, a large study from Australia found absolutely no difference between ICSI and conventional IVF in this regard.

In vitro fertilization achieves the highest pregnancy rates, compared with other assisted reproductive therapy (exceeding 50 percent in many centers), but it also carries the highest risk of multiple births and ovarian hyperstimulation, and it's expensive. It's used by only about 3 percent of infertile patients.

GIFT and ZIFT

Unfertilized eggs and sperm can be injected into the fallopian tubes through a laparoscope in the abdomen. This procedure is called gamete intrafallopian transfer (GIFT). The same procedure using fertilized eggs (zygotes) is called zygote intrafallopian transfer (ZIFT). These procedures are very rarely performed and are very expensive. GIFT achieves a pregnancy rate of about 30 percent, which has been surpassed by IVF in recent years. Because IVF is less invasive and achieves a higher pregnancy rate, GIFT and ZIFT are currently done only in unusual circumstances.

The Science
Behind the Scenes

t HIS CHAPTER IS for those of you who'd like to understand more about the science of this program, and specifically about the effect of insulin on the reproductive system. I didn't want to bog you down with too much medical explanation before you'd first understood the basics of my recommendations. If you're interested in learning more about the hows and whys of this program, read on. If not, skip ahead to Chapter 10 and I won't be offended.

The Purpose of Insulin

The hormone insulin, produced by the pancreas, is a key regulator for your body's energy needs. Insulin has had negative connotations lately because of the epidemic of diabetes, obesity, and the metabolic syndrome (also known as syndrome X), but in reality it is a very important hormone that does many good things.

Your liver produces a small amount of the simple sugar glucose, and the rest of your body's glucose comes from your diet. The body wants to have a constant level of glucose to feed the cells, providing them with energy. After you eat a meal, it wants to store the extra glucose for later use (when you're sleeping, for example, or between meals).

So, out comes insulin, a great multitasker. First, it signals the liver to stop making more glucose because there's plenty coming in. Then it "unlocks" the cells so that they can gobble up the glucose they need. Insulin cleans up the leftovers by making chains of glucose, called glycogen, because glucose is easier to store in chains. Then insulin shepherds the glycogen into cargo space in the liver and muscle cells. If you've eaten more than you need, it stores the rest in fat cells.

The hormone glucagon, also produced in the pancreas, works in the opposite way. When you're lacking nutrients or haven't eaten in a long time, insulin gets to take a rest. The body calls on glucagon to come out, blow the whistle, and bring the glycogen out of storage so that it can be broken down into glucose again and put back into the bloodstream. Glucagon can also signal the liver to make and release more glucose.

At least, this is how it all happens in an ideal world.

Insulin Resistance

Unfortunately, what often happens is that cells react to insulin the way unruly children react to a substitute teacher. That is, they don't listen very well.

Therefore, the careful instructions issued by insulin are not followed. Glucose doesn't reach the cells, so the body thinks there must not be enough insulin out there doing its job. It then sends out more and more insulin. But the result is too much blood glucose *and* too much insulin in circulation.

This is the phenomenon known as insulin resistance. The body is resisting—refusing to listen to the commands of insulin. If this happens long enough, the pancreas may give up producing insulin. That effect leads to diabetes.

The main difference between insulin resistance and type 2 diabetes is that when a person is insulin-resistant, the pancreas keeps producing more and more insulin to try to make up for its ineffectiveness. When a person is diabetic, the pancreas doesn't produce enough insulin to make up for the resistance.

Insulin Resistance: *Causes and Symptoms*

Insulin resistance has many possible causes. It does appear to be partly genetic, and people who are Latino, black, or Native American are more prone to this disorder. But the other possible causes are more subject to the chicken-and-egg question. We know that people with insulin resistance tend to be overweight, and particularly to accumulate fat in the abdomen. We don't know for sure whether insulin resistance causes the weight gain or the weight gain causes the insulin resistance. Most likely, it's a little of both: extra weight causes insulin resistance, which then makes it harder to lose weight, creating a vicious circle.

The more weight is gained, the worse the insulin resistance becomes. People with a BMI of 30 or greater have a fivefold greater risk of diabetes than people with a normal BMI of 25 or less.[1] The American Heart Association estimates that one in four people with insulin resistance will go on to develop type 2 diabetes.

(To calculate your approximate BMI, use the calculator at www.cdc.gov/needphp/dnpa/bmi/calc-bmi.htm. The CDC considers a person with a BMI below 18.5 to be underweight, a person with a BMI of 18.5–24.9 to be of normal weight, a person with a BMI of 25.0–29.9 to be overweight, and a person with a BMI of 30.0 or above to be obese.)

PCOS can cause insulin resistance. We also know that a lack of physical exercise aggravates insulin resistance. The condition is also associated with blood lipid imbalances: high LDL cholesterol, low HDL cholesterol, and high triglycerides.

Other signs of insulin resistance include high blood pressure, fatigue ("sugar crashes"), and carbohydrate cravings.

Most experts agree that lifestyle factors play a major role in the development of insulin resistance. That is why the condition is greatly on the rise as the American lifestyle becomes more unhealthy and sedentary. The more simple carbs (white bread, potatoes, pasta, bagels, donuts, and so on) we eat, the harder insulin has to work to deal with the high sugar spikes.

How Do Scientists Study Insulin?

It's not easy to evaluate and study insulin resistance. Much of the problem lies within the metabolism of individual cells and involves nutrients and metabolites that change in the blink of an eye. By the time the tissues are prepared for study, the components to be studied have changed or are gone altogether.

Recently, a technique called nuclear magnetic resonance (NMR) spectroscopy has opened a window for studying these factors noninvasively within living tissue. The technique is similar to using magnetic resonance imaging (MRI) to look at anatomy (for example, an injured knee or a suspected tumor); however, with NMR we can measure the concentrations of selected substances all the way down to the level of the individual cells.

Using NMR, scientists have made some fascinating discoveries about insulin metabolism.

Problems of High Insulin

Individual cells process nutrients and metabolites at different rates in different people. Your insulin metabolism—that is, how fast your body processes insulin—can affect many areas of your health.

High insulin levels cause the body to go into storage mode for a prolonged period of time. This causes potential energy, in the form of glucose, to convert to fat. The more fat there is, the harder it is to break down. And not only that—the higher the insulin levels and the more fat there is, the harder it is to get pregnant and the greater the chance of becoming infertile.

The body is a complex organism. Its systems are interconnected and interdependent. When something is out of balance in one system, it affects other systems, too.

Mitochondria

Recent research has found that individuals prone to insulin resistance and type 2 diabetes have fewer mitochondria than most people do.

Mitochondria are organelles—tiny parts of each individual cell in your body. Their main feature is a double membrane. The outer membrane is smooth, but the inner membrane is folded until it forms fingerlike projections called cristae. These cristae are where the mitochondria earn their keep by converting food into energy. Glucose combines with oxygen here to get broken down into ATP, the cells' main source of energy.

Normally, there are hundreds or even thousands of mitochondria in each human cell. When there are not enough mitochondria to do their job properly, the situation becomes like an assembly line with a missing person: things get backed up.

In the case of your body, the food your digestive system has broken down into glucose sits around in the bloodstream waiting for its turn to become energy. When too much glucose is stacked outside, the insulin shuttles the glucose away until the mitochondria catch up with production. Overflows of stored glucose become fat. People with poor mitochondrial function have higher levels of intercellular fatty acids, which hinder the enzyme functions involved in transporting and metabolizing glucose.

If the mitochondria never do catch up, the sustained high insulin levels and the extra fat can have a negative impact on your fertility.

Recent studies by the Mitochondria Research Society indicate that even sperm motility can be affected by mitochondrial function,[2] suggesting that mitochondria affect fertility in multiple ways.

Having too few mitochondria isn't as serious a problem as having, say, too few white blood cells, but it does influence how your body functions in the long run. It can have a domino effect on your body's systems, including your reproductive system. By making the changes I suggest, you will not only return to fertility but also live a longer and healthier life.

Testosterone

Testosterone is the major hormone responsible for turning boys into men. It is responsible for the growth of facial hair, a deeper voice, and the like. In adolescent and adult males, the testes produce it. But women's ovaries also produce small amounts of testosterone normally.

Testosterone exists in two different forms in the human body: bound and unbound. Testosterone binds with an androgen receptor, which interprets the testosterone for the person's genes. Unbound, or free, testosterone is loose in the bloodstream and is the form that exerts the biological effects.

Recent studies have found that higher amounts of insulin in premenopausal women stimulate ovarian testosterone production and result in higher levels of free testosterone in the system. High testosterone levels can interfere with the development of follicles, with ovulation, and with the production of cervical mucus. High levels can also lead to the development of PCOS.

PCOS does not occur naturally in Wistar rats, a specific type of rat used in scientific research that is intended to lead to better treatment of human patients. That is, polycystic-appearing ovaries do not occur in these research rats unless they receive daily injections of testosterone prior to puberty. When injected with testosterone, the Wistar rats' ovaries have developed cystic follicles, and ovulation has ceased.[3]

Luteinizing Hormone

High insulin levels lead to increased production of luteinizing hormone.[4] The pituitary gland produces luteinizing hormone, which is used to stimulate the production of sex hormones and incite ovulation. Too much luteinizing hormone signals overproduction of both estrogen and testosterone.

Insulin-like Growth Factors

High insulin levels also increase the amount of free insulin-like growth factors. These growth factors can inhibit the function of follicle-stimulating hormone (FSH), the hormone that tells the ovaries to grow follicles so that eggs can mature. Insulin-like growth factors and testosterone can both get in the way of this signal, raising the bar for how much FSH must be produced before a follicle develops. When there's not enough FSH to compensate, the follicles stay small and don't develop enough to produce an egg capable of being released and fertilized.

Follicle-Stimulating Hormone

In a study of insulin-resistant and non-insulin-resistant anovulatory women, researchers found that it took larger doses of FSH for longer periods of time to achieve follicular maturation and ovulation; and fewer of the insulin-resistant women conceived as a result of this therapy.[5]

In other words, if you have insulin resistance and you're not ovulating, your body will need to produce extra FSH or you may need to take medication that contains FSH to help your eggs mature. Even then, the odds of conception are lower than if you were not insulin-resistant, so curing this underlying problem makes a big difference. Further supporting this conclusion, several studies using medications to improve insulin production have found that it required less FSH, for a shorter time, to stimulate the ovaries in women who took these insulin sensitizers than in women who did not take them.

Follicular Atresia

When the follicle fails to rupture and release an egg, the follicle holding the egg degenerates and is reabsorbed by the ovary. The unreleased egg is lost. This natural process is called follicular atresia.

In the presence of insulin-like growth factors, the regression process is accelerated and follicular atresia happens more quickly.

The overall result, or culmination, of the chain of events—fewer mitochondria; backed-up glucose production; higher levels of insulin in the bloodstream; greater amounts of free testosterone; an imbalance among progesterone, estrogen, and luteinizing hormone; and high levels of insulin-like growth factors—is follicular atresia and the loss of the unovulated egg. So not only did you not ovulate during this particular cycle, but you may have lost fertile eggs that can't be replaced.

You need to break the cycle by controlling your insulin levels so that proper ovulation can occur. But not only does high insulin affect ovulation; it also has a major impact on implantation—the attachment of the embryo to the uterus—and thus can lead to a greater risk of miscarriage.

Isn't There a Pill for That?

Prescribing a pill is exactly what a doctor may do. Your doctor may determine that you need medication such as metformin or rosiglitazone to keep your insulin levels in check, and this is fine. But let's compare this to recurring stomachaches. Yes, there are medicines to treat an upset stomach; and yes, they can improve the condition. However, in the long run, it's better to treat the cause of the problem as well. Why are you getting so many stomachaches? Maybe you have a food allergy or are eating too much junk food or are under too much stress. Eventually, you'll want to treat these underlying causes, and the medication may become unnecessary.

At this stage, we must address not only the high insulin levels but also the changes they have caused in the way your body functions. If we correct them, the result is fertility. What I am suggesting is not a temporary fix but a permanent improvement in the way your body functions, and a better chance of becoming pregnant. Rather than just treating the symptoms, diet and exercise treat the cause.

At first glance, a surgical procedure may sound like a simpler answer than changing your lifestyle through diet and exercise. But there are risks in any surgery, and even the best fertilization techniques currently have a success rate of only about 50 percent.

I am not selling a get-pregnant-quick scheme, but I am offering a solution to your infertility that's risk-free and painless (aside from the occasional sore muscles from your new exercise routine). Mind you, although it may work in just a month or two, it may take longer. Several months may be required to get your insulin levels in check and your body responding properly. This program may eliminate the need for any fertility doctor, or it may become a complementary part of your treatment, increasing the odds that a surgical procedure or medications will work because your reproductive system will be in better shape.

Keeping Insulin Levels Low

The basis of my program is keeping insulin levels low. Numerous studies have found that low insulin levels improve a woman's fertility, increase her chance of becoming pregnant naturally, and lower the risk of miscarriage. Different doctors have used different methods to achieve lower insulin levels. Some have used prescription medication. Others favor weight loss and dietary controls.

Women who have used medication have had limited success in becoming pregnant without additional medical intervention. Previous research studies of weight loss did not study the effects of different diet plans on fertility; they studied only overall weight loss—or a single study compared similar diets without looking at the benefits of other diets.

A well-balanced diet, properly spaced meals and snacks to limit the time the body spends fasting, and a proper exercise routine are the keys to controlling rogue insulin levels and returning you to fertility without sacrificing your health or the fun of living life to its fullest.

Since I know you are curious, let's take a few minutes to look at what others have tried.

What About Medication?

As a result of diabetes research and other studies related to conditions characterized by high insulin levels, various medications are available to counteract the overproduction of insulin.

The most widely used of these medications is metformin, manufactured and sold under the brand name Glucophage. Metformin comes in tablet form and is taken orally. It was originally created for people with type 2 diabetes and is still widely used as a treatment for that condition. It must be taken with food or milk to prevent the body from absorbing the metformin too quickly. The exact dosage and the number of doses taken each day are determined by the doctor and depend on how high a person's insulin level is.

Women with PCOS were first given metformin to counteract their insulin resistance. When metformin is given alone, about 40 percent of women will begin menstruating normally, and more than half will show evidence of ovulation.[6]

When a woman with PCOS takes metformin combined with clomiphene citrate (the generic name of Clomid, a nonsteroidal ovulatory stimulant) for up to six months, she has a 70 percent chance of returning to normal menstruation and ovulation cycles and a 23 percent chance of becoming pregnant.[7]

Troglitazone, the generic name of Rezulin, has similar results. Like metformin, troglitazone was originally developed as a treatment for people who had type 2 diabetes, and it too is taken orally. It was designed to improve the insulin sensitivity of the body's muscles and adipose, or fatty, tissue. In one study, with troglitazone alone, 13 women achieved an ovulation rate of 42.3 percent (11 out of 26 cycles) after taking 400 mg. per day for 12 weeks.[8] When troglitazone was combined with clomiphene citrate (CC) therapy, the ovulation rate was 72.7 percent (8 out of 11 cycles). Clomiphene citrate alone achieved a 34.9 percent ovulation rate.

In studies related to fertility, up to 30 percent of women did not respond to the combination of clomiphene citrate and metformin, and more than 75 percent of the women in these studies remained unable to get pregnant. Such women have clomiphene citrate–resistant PCOS. Additional studies have investigated alternative pharmaceutical treatments for them.

One such study, conducted jointly by researchers in Egypt and Japan, examined the use of troglitazone. They found that troglitazone not only improved insulin resistance but also provided a reduction in the production of testosterone by the ovaries. In the opinion of the researchers, this was the key to its benefits in treating infertility related to PCOS. However, it also caused an increase in liver enzyme production.[9]

Because of the potential damage to the patient's liver, troglitazone is not approved for use in the United States. You don't want to play

Russian roulette with your liver. It's a vital organ. Presumably, you not only want to get pregnant but also want to watch your children grow up.

No prescription medications have been developed yet just to treat infertility related to insulin resistance. At this time, the only medications available were created to treat other conditions, such as diabetes, that are not related to fertility. The use of these medications to treat infertility arose out of doctors' attempts to treat the symptoms related to PCOS. Observation and research found that they could also help a woman regain her fertility.

Of the women using the most common medicinal treatment, a combination of metformin and clomiphene citrate, less than one in four will have a child using that method.

It's definitely an improvement over infertility, but I'd like to improve the odds, and that is why I have developed my plan to help increase your chance of becoming pregnant.

Diet and Weight Loss

One of the best methods of lowering high insulin levels is simply weight loss. Since the key to returning to regular menstruation and ovulation is reducing the amount of insulin in the body, weight loss is also one of the best methods of improving a woman's fertility. As little as a 5 percent to 10 percent reduction in a woman's weight can greatly improve her chance of becoming pregnant without expensive hormonal treatments, by improving insulin metabolism, improving androgen production, and permitting ovulation.

While others have conducted research into how weight loss affects fertility and have even examined current diet trends, little has been done to compare and contrast different types of diets and review various eating habits as they specifically relate to fertility.

The most extensive trial was conducted in 1998 by researchers in Australia. In this study, 67 anovulatory women completed a six-month clinical trial that focused on weight loss and fertility. In that time, 90 percent of the women resumed ovulating by the fifth month of the study. These women lost an average of 10 kilograms—a little over 22 pounds—and were still considered obese according to the body mass index (BMI), which doctors and scientists use to determine an individual's percentage of body fat.[10]

Of the 67 women who completed the study, 60 began ovulating spontaneously, 52 conceived, and 45 gave birth. Eighteen of those who became pregnant did so without any additional intervention once they lost weight. That is, more than 32 percent, or one in three, of the women became pregnant without medical intervention. An additional 40 percent were able to conceive with additional treatment by a fertility specialist. Both of these numbers are much higher than those achieved with metformin and clomiphene citrate alone, without regard to lifestyle interventions. Additionally, those women who did not conceive spontaneously fell into subgroups with other risk factors, such as smoking or a higher BMI at the end of the study.[11]

This study did not measure the methods used to achieve weight loss or the changes in insulin levels within the body. The dietary regimen was simply described as "healthy eating choices." As a result, it is difficult to determine from the data if the spontaneous pregnancies occurred because of the weight loss alone or as a result of improved insulin resistance.

I've found only one study that addressed pregnancy rates in women on a low-carb diet. In 1982, investigators in France had a notion that was truly ahead of its time. They gave oral glucose tolerance tests to 93 women with unexplained infertility, and found that one-third of the women had abnormal carbohydrate metabolism.[12] They gave all the women advice about a modified diet, but only 13 of the women followed the low-carb plan. All 13 women achieved a pregnancy spontaneously within six months.

However you lose weight, the loss will improve your chance of fertility. One of my patients, Ali Weiner, followed a Weight Watchers program and began exercising. She and her husband had been trying to have a second baby for two years.

"We thought it would be really easy because my son was an accident," she says. "When we decided to get pregnant, we figured, 'We'll just do it,' and then we started trying and it just didn't work."

Her son was already seven years old by that point, so she knew that the situation might have something to do with her age, but she had also been in better shape the first time. Ali began getting serious about losing weight in November, and she had dropped 16 pounds when she found out that she was pregnant in January.

Another interesting effect of weight loss, according to the French study, is an improvement in women's self-esteem. The women's anxiety levels and depression scores on standard psychological measures were reduced along with their weight.[13]

Why Didn't My Doctor Ever Tell Me?

Your doctor may not have mentioned that lowering body fat would help simply because he or she did not know. The research is still relatively new, and this treatment is still being explored. I am convinced that it will soon be the standard treatment for PCOS and for women with other, undefined fertility issues, just as it is the first-line treatment for problems such as high blood pressure, high cholesterol, and diabetes.

The actual amount of weight you need to lose depends on your starting weight. If, for instance, you weigh 200 pounds at the beginning of my diet, you would need to lose about 5 to 10 pounds of *body fat* to make a difference in your fertility. (This may translate into less overall weight loss as you improve muscle mass.) I would like to stress that this is an average weight loss, and that spontaneous ovulation begins at different times for different individuals.

Blair, from Rhode Island, wasn't even trying to get pregnant—in fact, she was taking birth control pills. Fertility wasn't on her mind when, at age 38, she began a lower-carb diet to lose weight. It took her six months to lose 80 pounds, from her initial weight of 278. She admits that she wasn't quite as diligent as she should have been with the birth control pills—she did forget to take them every now and then—but when she missed a period, she didn't think much of it. Her menstrual cycles had been irregular, sometimes coming every two weeks, sometimes skipping a month. But when she missed her period for two months in a row, she decided to have a pregnancy test. It was positive: she was nine weeks pregnant.

"I definitely blame my low-carb diet!" she says. "Let's just say we were flabbergasted. But here I am today, with a wonderful six-week-old."

Conversely, some women have too little body fat to ovulate properly. It is estimated that women need 17 to 22 percent body fat in order to maintain normal hormonal cycling. It is therefore common to see fertility problems in women with eating disorders such as anorexia or bulimia. However, such problems are not limited to this group of women. Competitive athletes may also encounter problems. Women with very low body fat typically have unusual eating patterns—so by following the meal schedule prescribed in this plan, they will be better able to achieve a more normal fat distribution and restore the hormonal cycle.

Carbs and Insulin

Several studies have compared the effects of restricted-carbohydrate diets and higher-carb diets with regard to insulin resistance.

Researchers in Italy put 10 patients on a restricted-carb diet (45 percent protein, 35 percent carbs, 20 percent fat) and 10 patients on a high-carb diet (60 percent carbs, 20 percent protein, 20 percent fat) for 21 days.[14] Then they measured insulin parameters with an insulin clamp and found that the women on the restricted-carb diet had improved insulin sensitivity, whereas those on the high-carb diet had worsened insulin resistance.

Another study found no difference in weight loss in two diet regimens similar to those in the study just mentioned; but only the low-carb diet improved insulin resistance, as evidenced by improved fasting glucose/insulin ratios.[15]

Finally, the Oslo Diet and Exercise Study, published in *Diabetes Care,* found improved insulin resistance with a low-carb, high-protein diet, whether or not the participants exercised.[16] The study also found a positive correlation between reduced insulin resistance and lowered BMI.

It has become increasingly clear that reduction in insulin resistance has a positive impact on ovulation and the ability to conceive and that this can be achieved through both dietary and medical treatments.

The dietary recommendations in my plan have been adapted from these and other studies demonstrating improvement in insulin sensitivity with ample intake of protein combined with limited intake of starchy carbs.

How Did Insulin Get Out of Hand?

One research study, conducted in 2002, looked at changes in human lifestyles from prehistoric times to the present. This study concluded that insulin resistance actually had advantages for survival and reproduction during the last ice age. During that era, humans consumed high-protein, low-carbohydrate diets simply because carbohydrates were hard to come by. When carbohydrates were available, the body stored the excess energy for later use.[17]

After the ice age ended, agriculture began and the consumption of carbohydrates increased; but because of how the carbohydrates—grains—were processed, only a modest amount of glucose entered the bloodstream. As milling made starches more digestible, insulin responses increased by two to three times compared with what they had been when humanity's diet consisted of coarsely ground flour and whole grains. Today, carbohydrates take even less energy to prepare and are more widely available, due to the explosion of convenience foods, such as sandwiches and fast-food meals. As a result, the body is storing energy for a time of future need that will probably not exist in the modern age.[18]

Evolution has played a role. Some traits that originally contributed to survival have become unnecessary and at times even problematic in modern humans. For example, consider wisdom teeth. They were necessary for chewing food in ancient times. Today, most people must have them surgically removed. We can hope that our insulin metabolism will adapt to modern needs sooner or later, but evolution does take time!

Miscarriage

Life is fragile. The beginning of life is even more so.

Regardless of any issues of fertility, approximately 15 percent of recognized pregnancies end in miscarriage. By "recognized," I mean that the pregnancy has been confirmed through a standard pregnancy test after a woman missed her expected menses. But the number of miscarriages may be much higher than 15 percent. Studies of the early stages of pregnancy suggest that up to 50 percent of all conceptions are lost, most of them before the woman realizes she is pregnant. In most of these cases, menstruation may appear to arrive a little late or to involve a particularly heavy flow. Some miscarriages even appear as normal menses.

After struggling to become pregnant, women with high insulin levels have a rate of miscarriage more than three times as high as the rate among women with normal insulin levels.[19] Women with PCOS, which is strongly associated with high insulin levels and insulin resistance, lose up to 70 percent of their pregnancies through miscarriage.

But with my help, we can level the playing field and improve your chance not only of becoming pregnant but also of carrying your baby to term. The good news is that by improving your insulin levels, you can also decrease your risk of having a miscarriage once you become pregnant.

Miscarriage related to insulin resistance is due to increases in the activity of many factors that affect embryo attachment. High insulin increases plasminongen activator inhibitor-1 (PAI-1). One of the effects of PAI-1 is to prevent clots from breaking down. Once clots form on the placenta, the oxygen and nutrients received by the fetus are limited. PAI-1 also hinders essential enzymes needed by the placenta and causes a less stable attachment. This results in miscarriage.

However, this condition appears to be reversible. Some pilot studies evaluating the chance of miscarriage after treatment with insulin-sensitizing medications have found remarkable reductions in miscarriage rates—in fact, a reduction to nearly normal. Other studies have found that lifestyle programs similar to our own have also succeeded in lowering the risk of losing a pregnancy.

This, in my opinion, is the most compelling reason to keep your insulin levels in check—not only while you're working on your fertility but also once you've achieved pregnancy. After trying so hard to conceive, you owe it to yourself to make sure that your pregnancy is as healthy as possible. Take care of the things that are under your control. That's your only responsibility.

Ten

For the Guys

*t*HE REPRODUCTIVE PROCESS works differently in men from that of women. Whereas women are born with all the eggs they'll ever have (about 400,000 to 500,000), men make sperm continuously—millions of them every day from puberty onward.

It takes roughly three months for each sperm to develop and mature, 74 days for it to go through several stages: spermatogonia, spermatocytes, spermatids, and finally spermatozoa. During the spermatid stage, the sperm develops its head, mid-piece, and tail while partly embedded in a protective Sertoli cell. When the sperm has gone through all its stages and is ready to make its exit, it is like a newly hatched bird: it has all the right features, but it's not ready to fly quite yet.

It still has one more trip to make: through the epididymis, a 20-foot-long curved, looped tube that makes up the outer structure of the testicles, where the sperm travels for about two weeks. Then it's better able to swim and ready to do its job, and it looks like a microscopic tadpole.

Before ejaculation, the sperm moves into one of the two vasa deferentia (singular: vas deferens), then through the urethra. If this mature sperm is not ejaculated, it eventually dies and is absorbed by the body.

Because of this process, it's important to note that any actions you take to improve your sperm profile may not be apparent for three months, the time it takes for new sperm to mature and gain the capability to fertilize an egg.

Factors Affecting Male Fertility

Male fertility is typically assessed by semen analysis. A man's likelihood of impregnating a woman is dependent on many things, but three main factors are evaluated:

1. Count (number of sperm present). A normal count is at least 20 million sperm per milliliter (ml.). Problems with sperm count may be identified as azoospermia (no sperm in the semen), oligospermia (not enough sperm in the semen, fewer than 20 million per ml.), or severe oligospermia (fewer than 5 million per ml.)
2. Motility (number of sperm moving forward). At least 50 percent should have progressive motility. Poor motility is known as asthenozoospermia.
3. Morphology (the shape of the sperm). At least 14 percent should be normally formed. Fewer than this is a condition called teratospermia. Irregular morphology includes sperm with an overly large head, two heads, or kinked or curly tails, for example.

Many factors can contribute to a low sperm count:

- Genetic abnormalities such as Y microdeletions, in which a piece of the Y chromosome is missing from the DNA.

- Anatomic abnormalities such as varicoceles (varicose enlargement of veins in the spermatic cord), congenital absence of the vas deferens (associated with cystic fibrosis gene mutations), or other obstructions anywhere in the long, complicated tract leading from sperm production to ejaculation.
- Hormonal problems such as low testosterone, low thyroid function, and high prolactin hormones.
- Neurological problems, which can lead to erectile and ejaculatory dysfunction.

A man with a low sperm count should see a doctor to assess the possibility of these abnormalities. Many are correctable and temporary, whereas others are permanent. However, in most cases there is no identifiable cause for a low sperm count. Sperm counts can fluctuate quite a bit over time, so a single test revealing a low sperm count doesn't have to be the final word.

Although more than 100 million sperm are typically ejaculated, only about 40 survive through the two-hour trip to the vicinity of the egg. Therefore, when the baseline number is halved, there is much less possibility that a single sperm will complete the arduous journey. However, it's likely that the quality (motility and shape) of the sperm is more important than the overall count. A sperm's job is to swim fast and straight. If it can do that, it has a chance of winning the race to the egg.

Other Potential Problems

- *Anti-sperm antibodies.* Sometimes a man's body can mistake a sperm cell for an unwelcome invader and build up antibodies to fight it. As a result, antibodies may attach themselves to the sperm, making the sperm clump together and causing problems with motility.
- *STDs.* As with women, certain sexually transmitted diseases such as chlamydia trachomatis or gonorrhea can cause scarring and obstructions in the reproductive tract.

- *Infections.* Infections can cause free radicals to build up and oxidize sperm cells and can cause scarring and swelling that harm the motility of the sperm.
- *Retrograde ejaculation.* This occurs when the urethra malfunctions and sends sperm backward into the bladder instead of out of the body. It may be caused by prostate surgery, diabetes, an injury to the spinal cord, or a number of other conditions.

Using the Program for Support

Male reproductive function isn't as directly influenced by insulin as female reproductive function is. Problems related to insulin can play a role, but typically only with overt diabetes; diabetic neuropathy leads to erectile and ejaculatory dysfunction.

However, the man plays an important role in supporting the couple's attempts at conception. By participating in the diet and exercise program, he will be better able to support and encourage the woman to achieve the goals and stay on track. The man will also be following standard medical recommendations for maintaining long-term health. There's no downside to men's participating in the same fertility program as women; while it's not likely to improve their own fertility, it is likely to help them feel great and become (or stay) healthy.

Supplements

Although many of the lifestyle interventions (diet and exercise) discussed so far may not be as directly applicable to enhancing men's potential fertility, there are a number of nutritional supplements that have been shown to improve sperm counts, sperm quality, or both. Some of the supplements are the same as those recommended for women; others are different.

L-Carnitine and L-Acetyl-Carnitine

L-carnitine is good for both male and female fertility, but for different reasons.

This amino acid is involved in shuttling long-chain fatty acids into the mitochondria for energy metabolism, and it helps transport toxic compounds out of the mitochondria. It's often touted as a supplement for athletes because it's purported to increase energy levels, burn more fat, and increase lean body mass. But what we're really interested in here is its effects on fertility.

The concentration of L-carnitine is nearly 2,000 times higher in the epididymis, where final sperm maturation takes place, than in the circulating blood.[1]

When seminal fluids are studied, L-carnitine levels are lower in infertile men than in fertile men. An evaluation of 79 men found that carnitine concentration in seminal fluids was positively correlated with total sperm count and the percentage of normal sperm forms.[2]

A problem related to L-carnitine can be treated with supplements. Studies have repeatedly found improvement in total motile sperm counts when men take oral carnitine supplements.[3] One group of 34 infertile men with prostato-vesiculo-epididymitis and normal seminal concentrations of white blood cells received L-carnitine and L-acetyl-carnitine supplements for three months; within three months of stopping the treatments, 11 percent of them achieved spontaneous pregnancies.[4]

Perhaps the best study on this matter was published in the medical journal *Fertility and Sterility* in 2004. This was a placebo-controlled double-blind randomized clinical trial in Italy, in which 30 infertile men were given 2 grams per day of L-carnitine and 1 gram per day of L-acetyl-carnitine, and 26 infertile men were given a placebo. Treatment continued for six months, followed by a two-month washout period.

The treatment group showed significantly improved motile sperm counts compared with the control group. All of this improvement was due to improved motility, not sperm production. Even though all the men had improved fertility after combined carnitine treatment, patients who had lower initial levels of motile sperm saw the biggest improvements.

The most substantial improvement was among the men who had started with fewer than 5 million total motile sperm. After treatment, their total motile sperm ranged from 3.4 million to 6.9 million, whereas the number in the control group ranged from 2.7 million to 3.4 million.

This is clinically significant because the average total motile sperm concentrations rose above the cutoff for a diagnosis of severe oligospermia (5 million). That changes a couple's therapeutic options from in vitro fertilization with intracytoplasmic sperm injection (IVF/ICSI) to intrauterine insemination (IUI); the latter is far less expensive and less demanding for the couple.

This trial substantiates the role of L-carnitine and L-acetyl carnitine in the sperm maturation process (as opposed to sperm production) and shows that these may be beneficial supplements for improving potential male fertility.

We recommend 2 grams per day of L-carnitine plus 1 gram per day of L-acetyl-carnitine, the amount shown to be effective in this clinical trial.

Carnitine is classified as a "conditionally essential nutrient." This term means that normally your body synthesizes enough of the nutrient, but you sometimes need more than your body makes. You can get about 75 percent of all the L-carnitine you need from a balanced diet. Good sources include red meat, dairy, fish, and avocados. You can also take it in supplement form: ProXeed is a citrus-flavored powder that dissolves in juice or other cold beverages and should be taken twice a day.

L-carnitine is not recommended for people who take doxorubicin

(Adriamycin, Rubex), isotretinoin (Accutane), valproic acid and its derivatives (Depacon, Depakene, Depakote), or zidovudine (Retrovir).

Mast Cell Blockers

Mast cell blockers are actually antihistamines, and several clinical trials have found that they can be effective in improving sperm quality. Mast cells are large connective-tissue cells that release histamine, heparin, and serotonin during allergic reactions or in response to injury or inflammation. Mast cell blockers are meant to prevent the ability of these cells to release inflammatory substances.

In 1995, a Japanese placebo-controlled single-blind clinical study enrolled 50 patients with severe oligozoospermia (lower than 5 million sperm per ml.). The patients received either 300 mg. per day of tranilast (a mast cell blocker) or a placebo, three tablets per day, for three months. At the end of the study, the treatment group had significantly higher levels of sperm density, sperm motility, and total motile sperm count. There were no differences between the groups in seminal volume or in normal sperm morphology.

Here's the important part: the pregnancy rate in the treatment group was 28.6 percent compared with 0 percent in the placebo group.[5]

In 2001, researchers conducted a second study with tranilast.[6] This time they chose 17 patients with a sperm density of less than 10 million, and gave them 300 mg. per day of tranilast for at least 12 weeks. Seven patients (41.1 percent) achieved significant increases in sperm count following the treatment, although sperm motility, semen volume, and normal morphology were unaltered. The important result? Three pregnancies.

It's certainly worth adding a mast cell blocker to your fertility regimen. However, the type of mast cell blocker or dosage or both may matter. A study in Turkey of 16 infertile men found no significant results or spontaneous pregnancies when the men took 180 mg. per day of fexofenadine (a different mast cell blocker, including the brand Allegra) for four to nine months.[7]

However, ebastine (another mast cell blocker) achieved positive results. In a trial of 15 idiopathic oligozoospermic males who received 10 mg. per day of ebastine for three months, nine patients (66.7 percent) showed definite improvement in semen quality.[8] The wives of three patients (20 percent) became pregnant within six months of the initial treatment.

Coenzyme Q10

Coenzyme Q10 is also a mitochondrial factor involved in energy metabolism, as well as an antioxidant.

It protects sperm from oxidative stress. Oxidative stress is a harmful condition that occurs when destructive atoms or molecules called free radicals accumulate and cause damage to a cell's components through oxidation, much as in the process that causes metal to rust.

In 1994, scientists in Italy found that in most cases, there was a positive correlation between the amount of coenzyme Q10 in a man's seminal fluids and his sperm count and sperm motility.[9] The only exception was in men with varicoceles, which is a varicose enlargement of the veins of the spermatic cord that produces a soft mass in the scrotum. (Varicoceles are common in infertile men. No one is quite sure why they sometimes, though not always, cause infertility, but the current theory is that they elevate testicular temperature too much. Corrective surgery is possible, but it doesn't always improve the odds for becoming fertile.)

For the men with varicoceles, there was no correlation between coenzyme Q10 levels and sperm motility. Also, they had greater quantities of coenzyme Q10 in their seminal plasma. During a follow-up study, the scientists found that men with varicoceles had slightly lower concentrations of coenzyme Q10 in the spermatozoan itself. This led the team to hypothesize that the protective mechanism antioxidants provide could be deficient in patients with varicoceles, leading to higher sensitivity to oxidative damage.[10]

Another study found that infertile men with low sperm motility, with or without varicoceles, had lower levels of coenzyme Q10 in their seminal fluids, as well as a lower ratio of the reduced form to the oxidized form.[11]

All this is well and good if it indicates an association between low levels of coenzyme Q10 and male infertility, but can we do anything about it?

Yes, according to a new study—the first treatment trial of coenzyme Q10 supplements on semen quality.[12] This was an uncontrolled pilot study of 22 infertile men with low sperm motility. They were treated with 100 mg. of coenzyme Q10 twice per day for six months. At the end of the study, there was a significant rise in their seminal coenzyme Q10 concentration (from 42 nanograms per deciliter to 127 nanograms per deciliter). More important, there was a significant rise in sperm motility, from 9 percent to 16 percent. When the men stopped treatment, their semen profiles returned to baseline levels two months later.

No change was noted in their sperm count or morphology, so if you know that these are your only problems, supplemental coenzyme Q10 probably won't help. But if the problem is motility, it does appear beneficial, and I advise the same dose used in the study (100 mg. twice a day).

Zinc

There is a high content of the element zinc in the testes and prostate.

Zinc is one ingredient of seminal plasma, and oligospermic men have significantly lower amounts of zinc in their semen than fertile men do.[13] Zinc deficiency can lead to lower testosterone levels and inhibition of spermatogenesis.

Zinc supplementation has been found to improve the sperm parameters of infertile men. In one clinical study, 100 men with asthenozoospermia were randomized into two groups: one group took 250 mg. of zinc twice daily for three months, and the other group served as controls.[14] There was significant improvement in sperm count, progressive motility, and fertilizing capacity, and a reduction in the incidence of antisperm antibodies, in the treatment group.

Lycopene

Lycopene is an antioxidant found in high concentrations in the testes and seminal plasma. Infertile men have lower levels of lycopene in their seminal plasma,[15] and this fact has led to interest in determining if lycopene supplementation could improve fertility factors.

Researchers in India published encouraging preliminary data about the effect of oral lycopene supplements on male infertility.[16] Thirty infertile men took 2,000 mcg. of lycopene twice a day for three months. Twenty patients (66 percent) showed an improvement in sperm concentration, 16 (53 percent) had improved motility, and 14 (46 percent) showed improvement in sperm morphology. Those whose baseline sperm concentrations were less than 5 million per ml. (four men) did not see significant improvements. Among the other 26 men, six pregnancies resulted (23 percent).

Vitamins C and E

Studies of rabbits and cattle have found improved sperm production with dietary supplementation of vitamins C and E; however, studies with humans have rarely shown the same success. Some metabolites actually worsen oxidative stress, so my advice is to ensure that you get the daily Recommended Dietary Allowance but not load up on either of these vitamins for the purpose of improving sperm counts.

What to Avoid

There are certain behaviors and risk factors that can harm male fertility.

Problems in the Workplace

A vast number of chemicals that men may encounter in the workplace can affect their fertility. To date, few of these chemicals have been studied in depth to find out just how much effect they may have; 4 million chemical mixtures in commercial use remain untested. According to the National Institute for Occupational Safety and Health (NIOSH), harmful substances can enter the body by inhalation, contact with the skin, or ingestion (if workers do not properly wash their hands before eating, drinking, or smoking).

REPRODUCTIVE HAZARDS FOR MALES [17]

Observed effects*

Type of Exposure	Lowered number of sperm	Abnormal sperm shape	Altered sperm transfer	Altered hormones or sexual performance
Lead	✓	✓	✓	✓
Dibromochloropropane	✓			
Carbaryl (Sevin)		✓		
Toluenediamine and dinitrotoluene	✓			
Ethylene dibromide	✓	✓	✓	

* Studies to date show that some men experience the health effects listed here from workplace exposures. However, these effects may not occur in every worker. The amount of time a worker is exposed, the amount of hazard to which he is exposed, and other personal factors may all determine whether an individual is affected.

(continued)

REPRODUCTIVE HAZARDS FOR MALES (continued)

Observed effects*

Type of Exposure	Lowered number of sperm	Abnormal sperm shape	Altered sperm transfer	Altered hormones or sexual performance
Plastic production (styrene and acetone)		✓		
Ethylene glycol monoethyl ether	✓			
Welding		✓	✓	
Perchloroethylene			✓	
Mercury vapor				✓
Heat	✓		✓	
Military radar	✓			
Kepone†			✓	
Bromide vapor†	✓	✓	✓	
Radiation† (Chernobyl)	✓	✓	✓	✓
Carbon disulfide				✓
2,4-dichlorophenoxy acetic acid (2,4-D)		✓	✓	

* Studies to date show that some men experience the health effects listed here from workplace exposures. However, these effects may not occur in every worker. The amount of time a worker is exposed, the amount of hazard to which he is exposed, and other personal factors may all determine whether an individual is affected.

† Workers were exposed to high levels as a result of a workplace accident.

To limit the risk of damage to your fertility from chemicals at the workplace, NIOSH recommends the following:

- Store chemicals in sealed containers when they are not in use.
- Wash hands before eating, drinking, or smoking.
- Avoid skin contact with chemicals.
- If chemicals contact the skin, follow directions for washing provided in the material safety data (MSDS). Employers are required to provide the MSDS for all hazardous materials used in the workplace.
- Become familiar with the potential reproductive hazards used in your workplace.

- To prevent contamination at home:
  - Change out of contaminated clothing and wash with soap and water before going home.
  - Store street clothes in a separate area of the workplace to prevent contamination.
  - Wash work clothing separately from other laundry (at work if possible).
  - Avoid bringing home contaminated clothing or other objects.
- Participate in all safety and health education, training, and monitoring programs offered by your employer.
- Learn about proper work practices, engineering controls, and personal protective equipment (e.g., gloves, respirators, and personal protective clothing) that can be used to reduce exposure to hazardous substances.
- Follow the safety and health work practices and procedures implemented by your employer to prevent exposures to reproductive hazards in the workplace.[18]

A further study by scientists in Italy checked up on the effect of traffic-derived pollutants on male fertility. They evaluated semen quality in 85 men employed at highway toll booths and in 85 age-matched men living in the same area, and found that total motility, forward progression, functional tests, and sperm kinetics were significantly lower in the toll workers than in the controls.[19] Stay away from those tailpipes!

Selenium

Selenium is a tricky subject: the fertility studies of this element are all over the map. What the research seems to boil down to is that neither end of the spectrum is good: high selenium and low selenium have both been associated with negative sperm parameters, including poor motility and low sperm count.[20] No optimal selenium range has been defined yet, so I do suggest avoiding supplements that contain extra selenium.

Smoking

Many studies have addressed the question whether smoking affects men's fertility. The answer? A resounding yes.

Smoking harms all areas of the sperm profile: count, motility, and morphology. A study of 655 smokers and 1,131 nonsmokers concluded:

> Cigarette smoking was associated with a significant decrease in sperm density (-15.3%), total sperm count (-17.5%), total number of motile sperm (-16.6%), and citrate concentration (-22.4%). The percentage of normal forms was significantly reduced in smokers, and sperm vitality, ejaculate volume, and fructose concentration were slightly but non-significantly affected.[21]

Even though male smokers' sperm factors still tend to be within normal limits, it's difficult to assess how much men's smoking affects the outcome of pregnancy—there are a few variables. If the female partner also smokes, her fertility is compromised. Secondhand smoke from the male partner may affect the woman's potential fertility. And several harmful components of cigarettes can pass through the blood-testis barrier and lower the chance of pregnancy.[22]

If that's not enough to persuade you to stop, smoking may also have a harmful effect on the developing fetus because of damaged DNA, and heavy smoking by the father during a pregnancy can increase risk of miscarriage.[23]

Marijuana and Cocaine

Marijuana use really does harm your fertility. It directly inhibits gonadotropin-releasing hormone (GnRH) in the brain, and this inhibition leads to low testosterone and low sperm production. The effects are usually reversible once marijuana use is stopped, but remember that it may take several months to see the reversal, because it takes about three months for a new sperm cell to develop and mature.

Cocaine use within two years of semen analysis makes you twice as likely to test positive for low sperm count. Those who've used cocaine for five or more years are more likely to show low sperm motility and a large proportion of abnormal forms.[24]

Anabolic Steroids

Use of androgenic steroids causes azoospermia (lack of sperm in semen), leading to infertility. Once popular primarily among professional weight lifters and bodybuilders, steroids have trickled down to high school athletes and casual gym-goers. This is bad news, because regular use of steroids can make it virtually impossible to achieve pregnancy.

The good news is that the problems with fertility are generally reversible, even among men who've abused steroids for a long time, but the reversal may take several months. According to one case study, a steroid abuser's semen was azoospermic at the beginning of the study period, was oligospermic five months later, and reached normal levels 10 months after the steroids were discontinued.[25] Other studies have found that it may take up to 20 months before semen profiles reach normal levels.[26]

Saw Palmetto

Saw palmetto is a commonly used herbal preparation for the prostate and is also marketed as an aphrodisiac and muscle builder.

It's believed to work in the prostate by blocking testosterone receptors, thus limiting enlargement. However, this antitestosterone activity can also hinder sperm production. For purposes of fertility, steer clear of saw palmetto.

There's a lot men can do to help or harm the chance of a successful pregnancy. Sometimes couples overlook the male role in fertility or miss the simple changes that may need to be made. You'll have a much better probability of conceiving if you're both following the guidelines in this book.

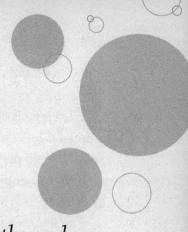

Eleven

Myths and Misconceptions

Myths About Infertility

It's a Woman Thing

One of the worst misconceptions is that infertility is a "woman's problem." Male factors are contributors in more than 40 percent of couples with delayed fertility, and are solely responsible for 20 percent of infertility. It's important for your partner to be tested by a fertility specialist or urologist—following this program to the letter isn't going to help if it turns out your partner isn't producing any sperm.

Even if you know you have problems with fertility, your partner should be checked anyway. You may both have factors contributing to infertility.

It Should Have Happened by Now

Even among couples who have no obstacles to fertility, when the woman is less than 35 years old, the normal chance of conceiving is only 20 to 25 percent per monthly cycle. After one year of trying, 85 percent of couples will conceive; after two years, 92 percent will conceive.

The chances decline slightly with each subsequent cycle during which pregnancy doesn't occur. If pregnancy hasn't occurred in the first year, the odds go down to less than 3 percent on the next cycle. That's why couples are called "infertile" after a year of trying. However, "infertile" (achieving no pregnancy in a year) is different from "sterile" (completely incapable of producing a baby). There are plenty of stories about couples who've restored their fertility after five or more years, beating the odds.

Megan is one of my patients who did just that. When she came to see me, she was 31 years old, of an average height, weighing 140 pounds, and she had gone through five years of infertility. Her menstrual cycles had always been irregular, and her basal body temperatures didn't show an ovulatory pattern. Laboratory evaluation showed that she had high testosterone levels. She started taking metformin but had to stop because of side effects. At the time, she was on no specific diet and exercised only very irregularly. Then she started on my program and took Clomid to help ovulation. She achieved a successful pregnancy on the first month.

Don't lose hope!

Wanting It Badly Enough

We may want to believe that successful women can accomplish anything once they put their minds to it—but with fertility, success is not just a matter of will. Most often, fertility has an identifiable cause, and overcoming it may not be wholly under your control. It may require medical intervention (for the woman, the man, or both).

There is also a clear decline in fertility with age. Before age 35, the likelihood of getting pregnant during any one cycle is 20 to 25 percent. By age 40, the likelihood is less than 7 percent per cycle. By age 43, it's less than 3 percent.

It's not wrong to build a career before building a family, but women need to know the effects of their age on fertility so they can make informed decisions for future planning. Many women don't find this out until they're in a fertility clinic trying to understand why they're having trouble conceiving.

Let go of any blame you may be placing on yourself or your partner. It won't restore your fertility or make anyone's life easier. Luckily, you're in a much better position than infertile couples of past generations; there are many interventions that may help. Educate yourself about your options. Take the actions that are under your control to improve your circumstances, such as following the recommendations for diet and exercise in this book and cutting out any contraindicated habits or supplements. Let go of the rest, because it's pressure that doesn't belong on your shoulders.

Magic Day 14

Women are often taught that they ovulate on the fourteenth day of their cycle (14 days after a period begins). Maybe, in a perfect world, but it's not all that likely in this one.

Day 14 is only an approximation, and it applies only if you have a model 28-day cycle. You can't depend on this calculation; it's much more important to chart your own fertility signals (basal body temperature [BBT], cervical fluid, and cervical position).

Sexual Positions

People often wonder if there are particular sexual positions that will help, or if tilting the pelvis upward after intercourse will help hold in the sperm. This isn't necessary, for various reasons.

The vagina changes its contour during intercourse to better hold the seminal pool in close contact with the cervix. It's documented that sperm take less than five minutes to travel from the vagina all the way through the tubes and into the pelvis. Therefore, the sperm are where they need to be before most people have finished having intercourse.

There's no harm in lying still for five minutes rather than getting up immediately, but it's not likely to make a big difference.

Side of Ovulation

There's a common belief that the side of ovulation alternates each month, left-right-left-right. It's actually totally random as to which side declares itself to have the lead follicle.

People who have one tube obstructed could potentially conceive on any given cycle.

Is Menopause the End?

Most people believe that the onset of menopause, either early or on time, renders a woman sterile. It is true that the likelihood of pregnancy is greatly decreased, but menopausal women may have as much as a 7 percent to 8 percent lifetime chance of conceiving. You may still ovulate even if you don't get a period.

One large study documented eight women out of 115 who conceived after they had met the criteria of menopause (no period in more than six months and a level of FSH greater than 40 milli-international units per ml.). More than half of the women had clear evidence of ovulation.

Sex Determination

People have cooked up a whole variety of techniques, rituals, and concoctions to manipulate the odds of having a girl or a boy.

Some of these methods are based on the fact that sperm containing a Y chromosome will produce a male, and the Y chromosome is smaller and therefore lighter than the X chromosome, which will produce a female. The actual weight difference, however, is so minuscule that it makes essentially no clinical difference.

Another pervasive myth about sex determination gained acceptance because it seemed to be rooted in science. Dr. Landrum Shettles, known as the "father of in vitro fertilization," published a method for predetermining sex by timing intercourse. It was based on where the woman was in terms of ovulation—intercourse three or more days before ovulation would increase the odds of having a girl, whereas intercourse closer to ovulation was better for a boy. This was not borne out in clinical studies; one study in New Zealand of 33 pregnancies concluded, "The results clearly refute the theory that intercourse close to ovulation favors male conceptions."[1] Several other studies followed, most of which concluded that it made no difference when the woman conceived. A few found a lower proportion of male births among conceptions that occurred during mid-cycle.[2]

The other suggestions from folklore are even less believable—sprinkle salt on your bed for a boy, eat chocolate if you want a girl, make sure the man climaxes first if you want a boy, have sex in the afternoon on an even day of the month before a full moon if you want a girl. Probably not surprisingly, none of these has passed the test of actual scientific proof. Deciding the sex of the baby is still Mother Nature's job.

Some fertility centers offer sperm sorting for sex selection; however, these utilize ultra-high-speed centrifuges to sort the sperm, and for the most part, they've had only limited success. Not all doctors will agree to use this method, for both professional and ethical reasons.

Cough Medicine

One piece of advice that's been circulating too long is that if your cervical mucus is too thick, you should take over-the-counter cough medicine to thin it. Cough medicine can indeed thin your mucus. However, it doesn't do a thing to improve your chances of a pregnancy.

Cervical mucus used to be evaluated by a postcoital test. The couple would have intercourse, then rush over to the doctor's office. The doctor would examine the cervical mucus, score it for a variety of features (ferning, stretchiness, etc.), and grade the motile sperm count within the mucus. This seemed to make sense—if the sperm weren't navigating the mucus, then they could not fertilize the egg. However, three studies found that pregnancy rates were identical whether no motile sperm were seen or the sperm received the highest score possible.[3] These results showed that the postcoital test was a waste of time, and it has since been eliminated from standard fertility workups. This also indicates that no significant effect will be achieved by improving cervical mucus. If the worst postcoital cervical score was just as likely as the best to be associated with conception, then measures to improve cervical mucus aren't going to accomplish much.

Feelings of Isolation

Many couples wonder, "Why is everyone else getting pregnant?" or "Why are we the only infertile ones?" The reality is that infertility is a common problem, affecting more than 9 million couples in the United States alone.

It's often useful to make contact with a fertility support group so that you can let your feelings out with an understanding audience.

Punishment and Faultfinding

Fertility and sexuality are morally charged issues. Often, infertile couples develop a sense of guilt because they feel they're being punished for moments of perceived moral weakness.

Infertility is nothing to be ashamed of, and it doesn't make you any less of a woman or man. Normal conception is such a complex process that it's a miracle that reproduction takes place at all! Clearly, it's common to have difficulty somewhere along the intricate chain of events that must take place. It's not designed as a process to weed out the immoral.

Stressed for Success

Some people will tell you that the reason you're not getting pregnant is that you're too stressed out. There's a funny thing about this myth: the more people say things like that, the more stressed you'll probably feel. It's stressful trying to get unstressed when there's seemingly so much riding on it!

There has been considerable research to determine if stress plays any role in fertility, and the outcomes have indicated that if stress plays any role at all, it's minor. Women typically don't feel stressed before they find out they're infertile; they feel stressed *after* they have trouble conceiving.

This myth goes hand in hand with the myth about adoption—that if you adopt, you'll suddenly get pregnant. The thinking behind it is that once you've adopted, you're no longer stressed about your fertility. However, this is erroneous thinking. We've all heard a story about a woman who got pregnant right after adopting a child, but those stories really are exceptions. The likelihood of getting pregnant after adopting is no different from the likelihood before adopting.

It's Rude to Question Your Doctor

It makes me sad that so many people are afraid or embarrassed to ask their doctors for information, clarification, qualifications, or success rates. Remember that the doctor works for *you,* not the other way around. This is an extremely complex field, and you should always feel free to ask questions.

Many of the tests and treatments are time-sensitive, so it's always better to ask and be sure of instructions than not to ask and potentially waste an entire month.

If you haven't succeeded with your primary doctor, ask for a referral to a reproductive endocrinologist. These are gynecologists who have completed several years of additional training to specialize in fertility problems.

Only board-certified reproductive endocrinologists are members of the Society for Reproductive Medicine and Infertility (SREI). Look for this seal on a certificate on the wall or in pamphlets in the doctor's office.

Special "Guy" Myths and Half-Truths

Boxers Versus Briefs

First, the logic of this one. It *is* true that sperm production is sensitive to temperature regulation of the testes. We know that acute fever will lower sperm counts, and problems like varicoceles that alter the thermal regulation of the testes are associated with low sperm counts. What we don't know is exactly how much heat, and applied for how long, will matter.

So the question wasn't unreasonable: Would brief-style men's underwear elevate scrotal temperature too much and lead to lower sperm counts? Lots of people assumed that the answer would be yes, but the clinical data failed to support popular opinion.

Researchers in New York checked 97 men and found that their usual underwear had no bearing on scrotal temperature, core temperature, or semen analysis, and that changing from briefs to boxers (or vice versa) didn't matter either.[4]

Saunas and Baths

Data on this subject are limited, but the sparse observational data that do exist show no effect from saunas on fertility levels.[5] Many doctors still suggest, though, that men trying to improve their sperm profile should not raise their scrotal temperature by taking long, hot baths or spending much time in saunas.

Bicycling

There has been rising concern about the potential effects of bicycling on fertility since health workers have emphasized physical activity for maintaining health. The question that's been raised is whether or not prolonged time in the bicycle saddle has a negative effect on sperm production.

It is clear that bicycling increases a man's risk for injury to the scrotum, and a study done in Germany in 2001 reported that 19 percent of male cyclists who had a weekly training distance of more than 400 kilometers complained of erectile dysfunction.[6]

But two clinical studies concluded that worries about cycling and infertility are probably overstated.

In 1996, researchers in Spain studied endurance athletes to see if their fertility levels were abnormal. These athletes included 12 professional cyclists. They were tested three times: in a training period, a competition period, and a resting period. Their profiles were normal, with one exception: they showed lower sperm motilities during the competition period. This finding was attributed to "physical factors associated with cycling, such as mechanical trauma to the testis and/or increased gonadal temperature."[7]

In a study in South Africa in 2004, researchers compared 10 cyclists with 10 sedentary subjects.[8] They noted no difference in sperm production or motility; however, compared with the sedentary men, the cyclists had a significantly lower proportion of sperm with normal morphology. The values were still all in normal ranges.

Pending further data from larger studies, it appears that prolonged cycling has little impact on semen analysis parameters. That said, it doesn't hurt to be careful. There are some protective measures you can take to reduce your risk of injury:

- Padded seats. Many bike manufacturers now make wider, more padded seats that are gentler on the perineum region.
- Padded shorts. You can also wear padded shorts to reduce the "shock factor."
- Proper position. Make sure your seat is at the proper height and angle.
- Limit yourself. If you're feeling numbness in the penis or scrotum, take breaks or cut short your training.

Lubricants

Most lubricants, even those marketed as "sperm-friendly," are *not* conducive to the survival of sperm. In a lab test, researchers observed what happened when sperm came into contact with K-Y Jelly, Astroglide, Replens, Touch, and two vegetable oil products. They reported, "Commercial lubricants inhibited sperm motility by 60–100% after 60 minutes of incubation. Sperm exposed to Replens or Astroglide were nonmotile and nonviable after incubation for 60 minutes, similar to the control, nonoxynol-9-containing product Gynol II."[9]

Saliva is also unfriendly to sperm. Allow time for foreplay, because the best environment for sperm is the natural vaginal secretions. If you must use a lubricant, the researchers found that canola oil had no detrimental effects.

Limiting Sex

Some people believe that men shouldn't ejaculate too often when trying to conceive—that it's better to store up lots of sperm so they'll be supercharged on women's fertile days. But you really don't have to worry about this unless you have very low sperm counts (in which case having intercourse every other day during fertile times is best). A man's body makes millions of sperm every day. You can have sex every day, and there will still be plenty of sperm racing toward the egg.

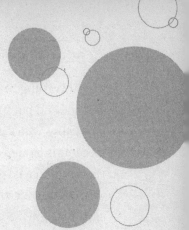

Twelve

After You're Pregnant

W HAT? YOU'RE PREGNANT? Congratulations! But wait—don't donate this book to the library just yet. There are still more things for us to discuss.

How Much Weight Should I Gain?

There's a wide range of what's "normal," but here's about what you can expect to gain by the end of your pregnancy. The numbers are based on your starting BMI.

WEIGHT GAIN DURING PREGNANCY[1]	
Starting BMI	Total weight gain
<19	28–40 lbs.
19–26	25–35 lbs.
26–29	15–25 lbs.
>29	15–20 lbs.

According to the Institute of Medicine, you should gain at least one pound per month, and no more than 6.5 pounds per month. You probably won't gain much during the first trimester—most of the weight is gained during the second and third trimesters.

Women who gain either more or less than these guidelines suggest have a higher risk of problems, including macrosomia (excessive birth weight), cesarean birth, low birth weight, and preterm birth.

The idea of "eating for two" is a bit overstated. Being pregnant doesn't give you a license to eat whatever you want whenever you want. A healthy pregnancy requires about an extra 300 calories a day to maintain—not an extra 3,000 calories.

Weight Distribution

According to the American Pregnancy Association, weight gain during pregnancy is roughly divided as follows:

- 7½ pounds is about how much the baby will weigh by the end of the pregnancy.
- 1½ pounds is how much the placenta weighs.
- 4 pounds is attributed to increased fluid volume.
- 2 pounds is the weight of the uterus.
- 2 pounds is the weight of breast tissue.
- 4 pounds results from increased blood volume.
- 7 pounds is attributed to maternal stores of nutrients and muscle development.
- 2 pounds is the weight of the amniotic fluid.
- Total: 30 pounds.

Losing Weight After Pregnancy

If you gain more than the recommended amount of weight during your pregnancy, you're likely to be overweight 10 years after you give birth.

Scientists at Gundersen Lutheran Medical Center in La Crosse, Wisconsin, examined 540 women through pregnancy, then six months later, and then 10 years later.[2] They found that those who gained the recommended amount of weight during pregnancy were about 14.3 pounds heavier than their pre-pregnancy weights 10 years later, whereas those who gained more than was recommended were 18.5 pounds heavier. There's a way to improve this situation— after the pregnancy, lose the weight fast! Women who lost all the weight gained during pregnancy by six months postpartum were just 5.2 pounds heavier at follow-up 10 years later. Aerobic exercise was a strong predictor of who would keep her weight down over the long term.

What Happens to Metabolism During Pregnancy?

Pregnancy is a relatively insulin-resistant state. The placenta produces human placental lactogen (HPL), a hormone that induces insulin resistance and carbohydrate intolerance and breaks down fats from the mother's body to provide food for the baby.

HPL can be tested to ensure that the placenta is functioning correctly. If the HPL level is too low, there's a higher incidence of preeclampsia (toxemia); and if the level is too high, there's a danger of diabetes.

An insulin-resistant state helps ensure glucose delivery to the baby, but it also predisposes women to develop diabetes—hence the routine diabetes screening.

A healthy lifestyle during pregnancy is very important for preventing the development of overt diabetes and helping you maintain a healthy pregnancy. Unfortunately, only one-third of women receive proper nutritional counseling during pregnancy. Between 40 and 60 percent of women have received no nutritional counseling during prenatal visits, and 7 percent have received incorrect guidelines.[3]

Dietary Recommendations During Pregnancy

Continue to eat balanced ratios of protein to complex carbohydrates at each meal. Ample protein intake has been found to produce a lower rate of stillbirths, neonatal deaths, and babies who are small for gestational age.

Diet and Morning Sickness

Plan to eat smaller, more frequent meals. Early pregnancy is often associated with nausea and vomiting (morning sickness, which women often say should be called "all-day and all-night sickness"). More than half of all pregnant women will experience nausea, and one-third will experience vomiting. This is due in part to high levels of human chorionic gonadotropin (hCG). No one knows exactly why hCG causes nausea, but the timing suggests that they are related. Generally, women begin to experience nausea just as their hCG levels rise during the first month of pregnancy, and the nausea abates as the hCG levels decrease around the twelfth to fourteenth week. If you're carrying multiples (twins, triplets, etc.), your hCG level is typically higher, and your morning sickness may be worse. Abnormally high hCG levels may indicate a molar pregnancy (a genetic error during fertilization that usually leads to miscarriage) or a tumor on the placenta.

Another factor in morning sickness is high progesterone levels, which slow the activity of the gastrointestinal tract so that the stomach empties more slowly than usual. This increases your stomach acids.

If you're experiencing nausea, you don't want your stomach to be completely empty or completely full—either state can aggravate the condition. This is why you'll want to eat several small meals throughout the day and night. As your uterus grows, it will compress the stomach, further limiting the amount you can eat at a single sitting.

Avoid fried foods and fatty foods, and limit dairy foods (try soy milk instead of regular milk). Spicy foods are definitely out of the question until you're out of the woods. Here are a few things you can try to combat nausea and vomiting:

- **Keep crackers by the bed.** Take your time getting out of bed if possible, and eat something bland before you get up. Crackers and dry toast are good options.
- **Use ginger.** Flat ginger ale, ginger tea, gingersnaps, shredded fresh ginger, and ginger candy are all possibilities. Ginger is well known for its antinausea properties. It has a strong taste, but if you don't like the taste, there are ginger pills available.
- **Get plenty of rest.** Lack of sleep makes nausea worse.
- **Carry a lemon.** Pregnant women can often be more sensitive to odors, and the unlikeliest smell may set you off. Citrus fruits, however, tend to calm queasiness. If you find yourself, say, in a smoky hallway, take out the lemon slices you tucked away in a little plastic container or bag and take a good whiff. They may help.
- **Drink fluids between meals instead of with meals.**
- **Wear motion-sickness bands.** These bands are best-known for combating motion sickness on an airplane or a boat, but they can be very effective against morning sickness, too. The bands press on certain pressure points on the inside of your wrist to prevent nausea signals from reaching your brain.
- **Take vitamin B_6.** The reason is unclear (pregnant women aren't typically deficient in this vitamin), but for many women, taking vitamin B_6 helps.
- **Get minty.** Peppermint is another food known to soothe nausea.

Try not to worry too much about morning sickness unless you're vomiting several times a day, you're becoming dehydrated, or you can't keep any food down. In your early pregnancy, your baby's nutritional needs are very small, and it's likely that you're keeping enough down to satisfy them. It's not unusual for women not to gain weight, or even to lose a small amount of weight, during the first trimester because of morning sickness. Ironically, morning sickness may be a sign of a healthier pregnancy: studies have found that women who experience morning sickness tend to have fewer miscarriages.

If your morning sickness is extreme, though, do see your doctor. You may have hyperemesis gravidarum, a rare but severe reaction that can last throughout your pregnancy and may need to be monitored. There are prescription medications available that are believed to be safe for pregnant women, including antihistamines and antiemetics. Of course it's ideal not to take any medications, but in a case like this, the potential damage to your health and the baby's health is greater than the risk of taking a medication to treat your symptoms.

Iron

Iron is an essential part of your diet during pregnancy in particular. You're at a higher risk of anemia, which can make you feel tired and look pale. Anemia makes it tougher for you to fight off infections and less able to tolerate hemorrhaging during childbirth.

Prenatal supplements should have enough iron in them to combat anemia, but iron may aggravate morning sickness. Do the best you can to get enough iron either through supplements or through iron-rich foods such as poultry, red meat, whole-grain bread, and enriched cereals.

Calcium

Pregnant women also need at least 400 mg. per day of calcium, which is 50 percent more than nonpregnant women need. You can get more calcium from dairy products (including lactose-free or low-lactose products). If you don't get enough calcium, the baby will start taking your calcium from your bones, leading to osteopenia (decreased bone density).

The FDA warns pregnant women not to take calcium supplements such as bone meal and dolomite, which contain a significant amount of lead.

Weird Cravings

Pickles and pistachio ice cream at 3 a.m. are among the odd joys of pregnancy. About 80 percent of pregnant women report having such food cravings. These cravings result from hormonal changes, not from nutritional deficiencies. However, it doesn't appear to be harmful to appease odd cravings as long as they don't severely disrupt your nutritional diet.

On the other hand, some women experience really weird, persistent cravings—nonfood items such as dirt, clay, chalk, soap, or starch. Some of these substances are toxic or are dangerous in some other way. Eating nonfood items is called pica, and this habit may be associated with iron deficiency. Tell your doctor if you're experiencing the urge to eat inedible substances. Typically, when anemia is corrected, the pica disappears.

What Not to Eat During Pregnancy

Warning: Avoid Mercury

Mercury poisoning causes a great deal of damage to your nervous and reproductive systems. It crosses the placenta and brain barriers quickly and has a long half-life (80 hours), so it slows brain growth and nervous-system development.

Even relatively low maternal levels of mercury are associated with developmental delays in children up to age seven.[4] The CDC estimates that 10 percent of women of reproductive age have mercury levels above those associated with neurological development problems.

The primary sources of mercury poisoning are fish and shellfish. While fish can be a good part of a healthful diet, pregnant women are advised to pay close attention to the types and amounts of fish in their diet.

The Food and Drug Administration (FDA) and the Environmental Protection Agency (EPA) revised their recommendations for pregnant women in 2004. They now state the following:

1. Do not eat shark, swordfish, king mackerel, or tilefish, because these fish contain high levels of mercury.
2. Eat up to 12 ounces (two average meals) a week of a variety of fish and shellfish that are lower in mercury.
   - Five of the most commonly eaten fish that are low in mercury are shrimp, canned light tuna, salmon, pollack, and catfish.
   - Another commonly eaten fish—albacore ("white") tuna—has more mercury than canned light tuna. So, when choosing your two meals of fish and shellfish, you should eat only up to six ounces (one average meal) of albacore tuna per week.
3. Check local advisories about the safety of fish caught in your local lakes, rivers, and coastal areas. If no advice is available, eat up to six ounces (one average meal) per week of fish you catch in local waters, but don't consume any other fish during that week.

Soft Cheese

Certain soft cheeses can become contaminated with *Listeria monocytogenes*, a bacterium that's very harmful to developing fetuses. This contamination causes the condition listeriosis. According to the CDC, pregnant women are about 20 times more likely than other healthy adults to get listeriosis, because of changes in the immune system that make them more susceptible to the bacterial infection. Signs of illness may appear a few days or a few weeks after infection and may include flu-like symptoms (fever, chills, muscle aches, and sometimes diarrhea or upset stomach); but they may be so mild that the mother doesn't notice them. Listeriosis can be transmitted to the fetus through the placenta even if the mother doesn't show signs of illness. This can lead to premature delivery, miscarriage, stillbirth, or serious health problems for the newborn.

Therefore, the FDA warns pregnant women to avoid the following:

Mexican-Style Soft Cheeses
- queso blanco
- queso fresco
- queso de hoja
- queso de crema
- asadero

Other Soft Cheeses
- feta (sheep's or goat's milk cheese)
- Brie
- Camembert
- blue-veined cheeses, such as Roquefort

Don't depend on your sense of smell or taste to determine if something is contaminated. Cheese that contains *Listeria* doesn't necessarily smell, look, or taste any different from uncontaminated cheese. Semisoft cheeses such as mozzarella, pasteurized processed cheese slices and spreads, cream cheese, and cottage cheese are safe to consume.

The FDA also recommends the following guidelines to avoid infection:

- Eat hard cheeses, such as cheddar, instead of soft cheeses during pregnancy.
- If you do eat soft cheeses during pregnancy, cook them until they are boiling (bubbling).
- Use only pasteurized dairy products. The label of such a product will state "pasteurized."
- If you do use hard cheeses made from unpasteurized milk, use only those labeled "aged 60 days" (or longer).
- Eat only thoroughly cooked meat, poultry, or seafood.
- Thoroughly reheat all meats purchased at deli counters, including cured meats like salami, before eating them.
- Wash all fruits and vegetables with warm soapy water.
- Follow label instructions on products that must be refrigerated or that have a "use by" date.
- Keep the inside of the refrigerator, countertops, and utensils clean.
- After handling raw foods, wash your hands with warm soapy water, and wash the utensils you used with hot soapy water before using them again.
- Do not eat refrigerated pâté or meat spreads. Canned or shelf-stable pâté and meat spreads can be eaten.
- Do not eat refrigerated smoked seafood unless it is an ingredient in a cooked dish such as a casserole. Examples of refrigerated smoked seafood include salmon, trout, whitefish, cod, tuna, and mackerel, which are most often labeled "nova-style," "lox," "kippered," "smoked," or "jerky." This type fish is found in the refrigerated section or sold at deli counters of grocery stores and delicatessens. Canned fish such as salmon and tuna or shelf-stable smoked seafood may be safely eaten.

Herbal Doesn't Mean "Safe"

The fact that something is labeled "all-natural" or "herbal" doesn't necessarily mean it can't be harmful. Mint tea, for instance, may contain pennyroyal oil, a toxic substance that has been linked with hepatic and neurological injury and death in infants.[5] It has even been used to induce abortions.

Other herbal substances with reported potential risks include sassafras, elderflower, black or blue cohosh, dong quai, feverfew, juniper, Saint-John's-wort, rosemary, thuja, and sage. Again, check with your doctor before taking any herbal supplements or teas.

Behaviors to Avoid

- *Changing the cat litter.* Try to persuade someone else to change the cat litter box while you're pregnant. Used cat litter can contain the parasite *Toxoplasma gondii,* which can cause toxoplasmosis infection, a rare but potentially fatal illness for the fetus. If no one else will do it, wear rubber gloves and a mask while changing the litter.
- *Hot tubs and saunas.* Although no reliable studies have linked hot tubs or saunas with poor effects on fetuses, cautious doctors still recommend that pregnant women should avoid getting too overheated. Warm baths are fine; hot baths are probably not a great idea.
- *Taking medications.* Even over-the-counter medications may be harmful to a fetus. Always check with your doctor before taking such medications. Don't assume that you can or can't take anything. Typically, women can stay on SSRI-inhibitors (prescribed for anxiety and depression) while pregnant, whereas Accutane (prescribed for acne) carries extremely high risks of birth defects. The antibiotic tetracycline is not recommended for pregnant women or young children because it can discolor developing teeth.
- *X rays.* Radiation is known to be harmful to fetuses, so any elective X rays should be postponed until after your baby is born. Low exposure to radiation may be necessary, though, if there is concern about a serious medical problem.

- *Removing lead paint.* You may already know that children are particularly susceptible to lead poisoning, which can cause developmental problems. The leading cause for concern is lead paint, which is now illegal, but if your house was built before 1978, you may have problems. Deteriorating paint from older houses can affect young children, especially because they tend to put their fingers in their mouths after touching things. However, removing lead paint yourself is not a good idea. If you try to scrape it or chip it off, you're likely to increase your exposure, because you'll cause dust particles to become airborne. Hire an expert for this job. Call 1-800 LEAD-FYI for a list of experts certified by the Environmental Protection Agency to inspect the house and soil for lead and remove lead paint.

Exercise During Pregnancy

There are many benefits to exercising during pregnancy. It can reduce backache, constipation, and bloating; improve your energy level, muscle tone, and endurance; and help you sleep better. It can even make delivery easier because you'll strengthen your abdominal muscles—the ones that are important for "pushing."

In addition, if you exercise during pregnancy, there's less risk of gestational diabetes, and you are less likely to need insulin if gestational diabetes does develop.[6] Some data also show higher placental and fetal weights if the mother began moderate weight-bearing exercising early in pregnancy or before pregnancy.[7] The increased weight would due to an increase in both lean body mass and fat mass.

In 1994, the American College of Obstetrics and Gynecology (ACOG) stated that women with uncomplicated pregnancies could engage in exercise without restriction, and that unrestricted exercise would not compromise fetal development. I urge just a few cautions, however.

In general, I recommend low-impact exercises because of the increased laxity of ligaments and the change in your center of gravity. During pregnancy, your connective tissues are softened to allow the pelvis to expand; however, this puts the rest of your joints at a higher risk of injury. Low-impact exercise (no jumping or bouncing) limits your risk of joint injuries and falls. Pregnant women in general, and especially those at risk of preterm delivery, should not engage in any activities involving the Valsalva maneuver (holding your breath and bearing down while exercising). This maneuver increases intra-abdominal pressure and blood pressure. If you have any obstetrical complications, make sure to consult with your obstetrician before starting any kind of exercise regimen. This warning applies to anyone with a history of heart disease, incompetent cervix, multiple gestations, second- or third-trimester bleeding, placenta previa, preterm labor, or preeclampsia, among other conditions.

Exercise Regimen

The CDC and the American College of Sports Medicine recommend 30 minutes of exercise on most days, even during pregnancy. The ACOG used to recommend that pregnant women monitor their heart rate to make sure it didn't rise above 140, but that recommendation has been withdrawn.

There have also been some concerns regarding the rise in core body temperature during exercise. However, this may actually lower fetal temperature by increasing uterine blood flow and skin vasodilation. According to the ACOG, there is no association between exercise, fetal hyperthermia, and birth defects.

Water aerobics are an especially good choice (under proper supervision) during pregnancy; water provides buoyancy to ease stress on joints and provides a thermogenic buffer, so that you don't get overheated.

Kegel Exercises

Strengthening the muscles of the pelvic floor is very important during and after pregnancy. The pelvic muscles endure a lot of weight and pressure from the developing baby, and a weakened pelvic floor can cause injuries during delivery, as well as problems with incontinence ("leaking," which is common toward the end of pregnancy and postpartum). Stronger pelvic muscles will help prevent these problems. In addition, strengthened pelvic muscles can improve your sex life, increasing the pleasure for both you and your partner.

Kegels strengthen your pubococcygeal (PC) muscles and thus benefit your urethra, bladder, uterus, and rectum. They're simple to do and can be done anywhere—sitting, lying down, standing, in the office, in your car. No one will ever know. You can also practice Kegels during sex. Of course, then someone *will* know, but it'll probably be a welcome activity!

To get the feel for this exercise, next time you use the toilet, try to stop the flow of urine. Feel those muscles? Those are the ones you want to work on. You can practice by starting and stopping the flow of urine a few times; then, once you get the hang of it, you'll know what the exercise feels like and you can do it anywhere you choose.

About 25 times a day to start, building up to 100 times a day, contract those muscles and hold the contraction for 3 to 5 seconds, then release it. You should feel as if you're trying to pull your pelvic muscles upward toward your belly button. As you build the muscles, you should be able to hold the contraction for longer periods of time and do more repetitions.

Adding vaginal cones to your Kegel routine can significantly strengthen your pelvic-floor muscles.[8]

Try to keep up this exercise not only during pregnancy but also afterward. Keeping those muscles tightened lowers your risk of hemorrhoids and incontinence at any stage of your life. It's no fun worrying about "leaking" every time you cough or sneeze.

Pelvic Tilts

Another important exercise during pregnancy is the pelvic tilt, which strengthens your back and abdomen, lessening back pain and strain.

To complete this exercise:

1. Lie on your back with knees bent, feet shoulder-width apart, and heels on the floor.
2. Tighten your abdominal and gluteus muscles.
3. Press the small of your back against the floor (or mat), tilting your pelvis slightly upward.
4. Hold for 10 seconds, then relax.

Repeat this exercise several times. You can also try a different version of pelvic tilts:

1. Get on your hands and knees, arms outstretched.
2. Relax your lower back. You should feel that it's dipped (arched) slightly inward.
3. Now straighten your back by tilting the pelvis, trying to make it perfectly flat (not rounded upward).
4. Hold for 10 seconds, then relax.

Activities Not to Do During Pregnancy

- Scuba diving is generally not recommended. Diving below 30 feet is associated with a threefold increase in miscarriage and birth defects, as well as higher rates of growth restriction and preterm delivery.

- Horseback riding.
- Heavy weight lifting.
- Anything that requires you to change direction quickly.

Drink Your Water

Of course, you should drink eight glasses of water a day whether you're pregnant or not, but this is even more important when you're pregnant. It's easy for you to get dehydrated while you're pregnant, and dehydration can lead to a host of problems. The less serious consequences include fatigue, headaches, and dry skin. The very serious consequences include a risk of toxemia, poor removal of fetal waste, urinary infections, low amniotic fluids (oligohydramnios), anxiety, and depression.

While eight glasses (64 ounces) of water per day is a good estimation of the minimum your body needs, it's not enough for everyone. Women who exercise during pregnancy and women who are overweight often need more water, for example; and if you consume caffeine (coffee, tea, etc.), you'll need more water to combat its fluid-leeching effects.

The color of your urine is a strong indicator of whether or not you're getting enough water. The darker the color, the more dehydrated you may be. Ideally, your urine should be a very light yellow or nearly clear. If it's not, more water is in order. Try to carry a water bottle at all times, and write down your water intake to get a clear picture of how much you're drinking. You really can't overdo it with water, so drink as much as you possibly can.

Plan Summary

So there you have it! You now have all the tools you need to improve your fertility. Here's a quick reminder of the basic steps to follow.

Diet

Eat three meals a day and two snacks. One of the snacks should be eaten close to bedtime. Determine your daily protein needs; then get an equal number of grams of protein and carbs in each of your meals and snacks, and half that amount of fat. Limit starchy carbs. Plan ahead: prepare meals and snacks to take with you when you're on the go.

Supplements

Begin taking a prenatal vitamin.

Exercise

Get aerobic exercise five to six times a week (30 minutes each time) and resistance exercise twice a week, or do circuit training five to six days a week.

Journal

Write down all your food choices (with nutritional contents noted) and all the exercise you've done.

Emotional Support

Find a therapist or support group if you like. Make sure that you have a "fertility partner" to report to. Nurture your relationship with your significant other.

Additional Resources

American College of Obstetricians and Gynecologists (ACOG) Resource Center
Phone: (800) 762-2264, ext. 192 (for publications requests only)
Website: www.acog.org

American Society for Reproductive Medicine
Phone: (205) 978-5000
Website: www.asrm.org

Food and Drug Administration (FDA)
Phone: (888) 463-6332
Website: www.fda.gov

InterNational Council on Infertility Information Dissemination, Inc.
Phone: (703) 379-9178
Website : www.inciid.org

National Women's Health Information Center (NWHIC)
Phone: (800) 994-9662
Website: www.4woman.gov

Resolve: The National Infertility Association
Phone: (617) 623-0744
Website: www.resolve.org

Glossary

Adhesion: Scarring as a result of tissue injury from infections, surgery, or endometriosis that can lead to infertility. May be treatable through laparoscopic surgery if mild.

Amenorrhea: Lack of a menstrual period. It's called primary amenorrhea if the woman has never menstruated, and secondary amenorrhea if she menstruated in the past but hasn't had a period in at least six months.

Amino acids: Twenty kinds of molecules that link together in long chains to form proteins. A nonessential amino acid is one that the human body is capable of making on its own. An essential amino acid is one that we have to get from our diet.

Androgens: Male sex hormones.

Anovulation: Lack of ovulation.

ART: Acronym for assisted reproductive technology; a catchall term for medically assisted conception.

Artificial insemination (AI): Process by which sperm is injected into the cervix or uterus with a catheter attached to a syringe.

Asthenozoospermia: Low sperm motility.

Azoospermia: Lack of sperm in the semen due to a testicular malfunction or blockage in the reproductive tract.

Basal body temperature (BBT): Used to predict ovulation, a measurement of body temperature at its lowest point, usually checked right after awakening. BBT typically rises half a degree during ovulation.

Beta hCG test: Blood test to detect early stages of pregnancy by checking levels of a hormone produced by the embryo.

Clomiphene citrate: Synthetic selective estrogen receptor modulator (SERM) tablets used to induce ovulation.

Dysmenorrhea: Painful menstruation that causes cramping, bloating, or backaches.

Ectopic pregnancy: Condition in which an embryo is implanted outside the uterus, usually in the fallopian tubes, ovaries, cervix, or abdomen.

Embryo transfer: Process by which an egg fertilized in a laboratory is inserted into a woman's uterus.

Endometriosis: Presence and growth of endometrial tissue (which belongs in the uterus) outside the uterus, usually in other areas of a woman's reproductive tract. This disorder may be asymptomatic or may cause severe pelvic pain. It often causes infertility.

Epididymis: Long, coiled tube attached to the back of the testes. Sperm finish their maturation process here.

Estrogen: Female sex hormone.

Fallopian tubes: Tubes connecting the ovary to the uterus; normally the location where a sperm fertilizes an egg.

Fecundity: Likelihood of becoming pregnant in any one menstrual cycle.

Fetus: Term for a baby as it develops in the womb from eight weeks to full term.

Follicle: Fluid-filled cluster of cells inside the ovary where an egg develops.

Follicle-stimulating hormone (FSH): Hormone produced by the pituitary gland. In women, this hormone helps the egg to mature while in a follicle. In men, it stimulates sperm growth.

Follicular phase: Preovulatory portion of a woman's menstrual cycle. In a normal cycle, several follicles begin to develop during this phase, but only a single egg is released during ovulation.

Free radical: Highly reactive atom or group of atoms having one or more unpaired electrons. Can cause damage to cells and accelerate disease.

Hirsutism: Excessive body hair, often seen in women with PCOS.

Hypoestrogenic: Having a level of estrogen that is lower than normal.

Hypospermatogenesis: Low sperm production.

Hypothalamus: The part of the brain that controls (among other things) ovulation and the production of sex hormones.

Intracytoplasmic sperm injection (ICSI): Process in assisted reproduction in which a single sperm is injected into an egg.

In vitro fertilization: Process in which eggs and sperm are combined for fertilization in a laboratory dish instead of within the woman's body.

Infertility: Inability to conceive after frequent unprotected sex for one year.

The condition is called secondary infertility when a person has successfully achieved pregnancy in the past but now cannot.

Luteal phase: Postovulatory phase of a woman's menstrual cycle when the ovary produces progesterone.

Luteinizing hormone: Hormone that triggers the ovarian follicle to release a mature egg and begin ovulation.

Microdeletion: Mutation in which a piece of a chromosome is missing.

Oligomenorrhea: Infrequent menstrual periods.

Oligozoospermia: Low sperm count (below 20 million per ml. of semen).

Oocyte: Scientific term for the female gamete, usually referred to as the egg.

Ovarian hyperstimulation syndrome: Side effect of treatments that stimulate ovulation; it can occur when too many eggs are produced and a woman's ovaries become enlarged. Rarely, severe forms can lead to metabolic abnormalities and may be potentially life-threatening.

Oviduct: Another word for fallopian tube.

Ovulation: Release of an egg from the ovarian follicle.

Polycystic ovary syndrome (PCOS): Condition defined by the presence of any two of three diagnostic criteria: chronic anovulation, excess androgen production, and polycystic-appearing ovaries on ultrasound. A frequent cause of infertility.

Progesterone: Hormone produced by the ovary after ovulation to cause the uterus to prepare its lining to protect a pregnancy.

Retrograde ejaculation: Condition in which sperm are pushed backward into the bladder instead of out through the urethra.

Semen: Also known as seminal fluid, this is the ejaculated material. It includes sperm and secretions from the prostate, the seminal vesicles, and the vasa deferentia.

Sperm antibodies: Agents that may be present in a man's body and react against his own sperm; or agents present in a woman's body that "fight off" incoming sperm. These are antibodies from the immune system that mistakenly attack and harm sperm.

Spontaneous abortion: Pregnancy lost in the first 20 weeks. This is what doctors usually call a miscarriage.

Umbilical cord: Cord containing a vein and two arteries that connect a fetus to the placenta, the source of nutrients and oxygen.

Uterus: Womb. This is the organ that supports a fetus.

Varicocele: Enlarged or twisted vein in the scrotum that may lead to problems with fertility.

Vas deferens: Tube though which sperm travel from the epididymis to the urethra.

Zygote: Fertilized egg that hasn't yet divided.

Zygote intrafallopian transfer (ZIFT): Fertility technique in which eggs are harvested from a woman's ovaries and fertilized with sperm in a laboratory. The zygotes are then inserted into the woman's fallopian tubes.

Chapter 1

1. "Infertility Facts," fact sheet from the American Fertility Association, 2005.

2. "Age and Fertility," American Society for Reproductive Medicine Patient Information Series, 2003.

3. Seymour, et al., "A Case of Authenticated Fertility in a Man of 94," *Journal of the American Medical Association* 423 (1935).

4. L. Johnson, et al., "Influence of Age on Sperm Production and Testicular Weights in Men," *Journal of Reproduction and Fertility* 70, no. 1 (1984): 211–218.

5. K. M. Flegal, et al., "Prevalence and Trends in Obesity among U.S. Adults, 1999–2000," *Journal of the American Medical Association* 288 (2002): 1723–1727.

6. "STDs in Women and Infants," STD Surveillance Report 2000; National Center for HIV, STD, and TB Prevention; Centers for Disease Control and Prevention.

7. Ibid.

8. Ibid.

9. S. Wild, et al., "Global Prevalence of Diabetes: Estimates for the Year 2000 and Projections for 2030," *Diabetes Care* 27, no. 5 (May 2004): 1047–1053.

10. Piatti, et al., "Hypocaloric High-Protein Diet Improves Glucose Oxidation and Spares Lean Body Mass: Comparison to Hypocaloric High-Carbohydrate Diet," *Metabolism* 43, no. 12 (December 1994): 1481–1487.

11. Golay, et al., "Weight Loss with Low or High Carbohydrate Diet?" *International Journal of Obesity and Related Metabolic Disorders* 20, no. 12 (December 1996): 1067–1072.

Chapter 2

1. *Recommended Dietary Allowances,* 10th ed., Subcommittee on the Tenth Edition of the Recommended Dietary Allowances, Food and Nutrition Board, Commission on Life Sciences, National Research Council (1989).

2. D. Feskanich, et al., "Protein Consumption and Bone Fractures in Women," *American Journal of Epidemiology* 143, no. 5 (March 1, 1996): 472–479.

3. U.S. Department of Agriculture (USDA) National Nutrient Database, Release 17.

4. "High Protein Diet May Be Bad for Women Trying to Conceive" (press release), European Society for Human Reproduction and Embryology (June, 2004). (See www.eshre.com/emc.asp?pageId=459.)

5. "Dietary Reference Intakes for Vitamin C, Vitamin E, Selenium, and Carotenoids," Food and Nutrition Board, National Academy of Sciences, (August 2000).

6. R. M. van Dam, et al., "Coffee Consumption and Incidence of Impaired Fasting Glucose, Impaired Glucose Tolerance, and Type 2 Diabetes: The Hoorn Study," *Diabetologia* 47, no. 12 (December 2004): 2152–2159.

7. S. Lee, et al., "Caffeine Ingestion Is Associated with Reductions in Glucose Uptake Independent of Obesity and Type 2 Diabetes Before and After Exercise Training," *Diabetes Care* 28, no. 3 (March 2005): 566–572.

8. Raloff, "Coffee, Spices, Wine: New Dietary Ammo Against Diabetes?" *Science News* (May 1, 2004).

9. A. Wilcox, et al., "Caffeinated Beverages and Decreased Fertility," *Lancet* 2, nos. 8626–8627 (December 24–31, 1988): 1453–1456.

10. U.S. Food and Drug Administration and National Soft Drink Association.

Chapter 4

1. Dunstan, et al., "High-Intensity Resistance Training Improves Glycemic Control in Older Patients with Type 2 Diabetes," *Diabetes Care* 25, no. 10 (October 2002): 1729–1736.

Chapter 5

1. B. B. Qi and K. E. Dennis, "The Adoption of Eating Behaviors Conducive to Weight Loss," *Eating Behaviors* 1, no. 1 (September 2000): 23–31.

2. J. Wylie-Rosett, et al., "Computerized Weight Loss Intervention Optimizes Staff Time: The Clinical and Cost Results of a Controlled Clinical Trial Conducted in a Managed Care Setting," *Journal of the American Dietetic Association* 101, no. 10 (October 2001): 1155–1162.

3. R. C. Baker and D. S. Kirschenbaum, "Weight Control During the Holidays: Highly Consistent Self-Monitoring as a Potentially Useful Coping Mechanism," *Health Psychology* 17, no. 4 (July 1998): 367–370.

Chapter 6

1. Elisabeth Kübler-Ross, *On Death and Dying* (New York: Scribner, 1997). Originally published 1969.

2. R. Roopnarinesingh, et al., "An Assessment of Mood in Males Attending an Infertility Clinic," *Irish Medical Journal* 97, no. 10 (November–December 2004): 310–311.

3. L. K. Dhaliwal, et al., "Psychological Aspects of Infertility Due to Various Causes—Prospective Study," *International Journal of Fertility and Women's Medicine* 49, no. 1 (January–February 2004): 44–48.

4. "2002 Assisted Reproductive Technology (ART) Report," CDC Division of Reproductive Health.

Chapter 7

1. D. S. Lamson and S. M. Plaza, "The Safety and Efficacy of High-Dose Chromium," *Alternative Medicine Review* 7, no. 3 (June 2002): 218–235.

2. A. De Gaetano, et al., "Carnitine Increases Glucose Disposal in Humans," *Journal of the American College of Nutrition* 18, no. 4 (August 1999): 289–295.

3. S. S. Shankar, et al., "L-carnitine May Attenuate Free Fatty Acid–Induced Endothelial Dysfunction," *Annals of the New York Academy of Science* 1033 (November 2004): 189–197.

4. A. M. Fulghesu, et al., "N-Acetyl-Cysteine Treatment Improves Insulin Sensitivity in Women with Polycystic Ovary Syndrome," *Fertility and Sterility* 77, no. 6 (June 2002) 1128–1135.

5. A. Y. Rizk, et al., "N-Acetyl-Cysteine Is a Novel Adjuvant to Clomiphene Citrate in Clomiphene Citrate–Resistant Patients with Polycystic Ovary Syndrome," *Fertility and Sterility* 83, no. 2 (February 2005): 367–370.

6. S. Jacob, et al., "Oral Administration of RAC-Alpha-Lipoic Acid Modulates Insulin Sensitivity in Patients with Type-2 Diabetes Mellitus: A Placebo-Controlled Pilot Trial," *Free Radical Biology and Medicine* 27, nos. 3–4 (August 1999): 309–314. See also S. Jacob, et al., "Improvement of Insulin-Stimulated Glucose-Disposal in Type 2 Diabetes After Repeated Parenteral Administration of Thioctic Acid," *Experimental and Clinical Endocrinology and Diabetes* 104, no. 3 (1996): 284–288.

7. D. W. Lamson and S. M. Plaza, "Mitochondrial Factors in the Pathogenesis of Diabetes: A Hypothesis for Treatment," *Alternative Medicine Review* 7, no. 2 (April 2002): 94–111.

8. R. B. Singh, et al., "Effect of Hydrosoluble Coenzyme Q10 on Blood Pressures and Insulin Resistance in Hypertensive Patients with Coronary Artery Disease," *Journal of Human Hypertension* 13, no. 3 (March 1999): 203–208.

9. A. Lewin and H. Lavon, "The Effect of Coenzyme Q10 on Sperm Motility and Function," *Molecular Aspects of Medicine* 18, suppl. (1997): S213–S219.

10. K. Sekiya, et al., "Enhancement of Insulin Sensitivity in Adipocytes by Ginger," *Biofactors* 22, nos. 1–4 (2004): 153–156.

11. E. A. Sotaniemi, et al., "Ginseng Therapy in Non-Insulin-Dependent Diabetic Patients," *Diabetes Care* 18, no. 10 (October 1995): 1373–1375.

12. A. S. Attele, et al., "Antidiabetic Effects of Panax Ginseng Berry Extract and the Identification of an Effective Component," *Diabetes* 51, no. 6 (June 2005): 1851–1858. See Also V. Vuksan, et al., "Konjac-Mannan and American Ginseng: Emerging Alternative Therapies for Type 2 Diabetes Mellitus," *Journal of the American College of Nutrition* 20, no. 5, suppl. (October 2001): 370S–380S.

13. C. L. Broadhurst, et al., "Insulin-Like Biological Activity of Culinary and Medicinal Plant Aqueous Extracts in Vitro," *Journal of Agricultural and Food Chemistry* 48, no. 3 (March 2000): 849–852.

14. M. Q. Husein and R. T. Kridli, "Reproductive Responses Following Royal Jelly Treatment Administered Orally or Intramuscularly into Progesterone-Treated Awassi Ewes," *Animal Reproduction Science* 74, nos. 1–2 (November 15, 2002): 45–53.

15. H. Tsuneki, et al., "Effect of Green Tea on Blood Glucose Levels and Serum Proteomic Patterns in Diabetic (db/db) Mice and on Glucose Metabolism in Healthy Humans," *BMC Pharmacology* 4, no. 1 (August 26, 2004): 18.

16. Charles Choi, "Tea Gives Big Boost to Insulin," United Press International (October 10, 2002).

17. J. W. Anderson, "Dietary Fiber and Diabetes: A Comprehensive Review and Practical Application," *Journal of the American Dietetic Association* 87, no. 9 (September 1987): 1189–1197.

18. A. D. Liese, et al., "Whole-Grain Intake and Insulin Sensitivity: The Insulin Resistance Atherosclerosis Study," *American Journal of Clinical Nutrition* 78, no. 5 (November 2003): 965–971.

19. J. M. Kawa, C. G. Taylor, and R. Przybylski, "Buckwheat Concentrate Reduces Serum Glucose in Streptozotocin-Diabetic Rats," *Journal of Agricultural and Food Chemistry* 51, no. 25 (December 3, 2003): 7287–7291.

20. M. J. Iuorno, et al., "Effects of D-Chiro-Inositol in Lean Women with the Polycystic Ovary Syndrome," *Endocrine Practice* 8, no. 6 (November–December 2002): 417–423.

21. A. Khan, et al., "Insulin Potentiating Factor and Chromium Content of Selected Foods and Spices," *Biological Trace Element Research* 24, no. 3 (March 1990): 183–188.

22. Ibid.

23. R. Chang, P. H. Chung, and Z. Rosenwaks, "Role of Acupuncture in the Treatment of Female Infertility," *Fertility and Sterility* 78, no. 6 (December 2002): 1149–1153.

24. E. Stener-Victorin, et al., "Effects of Electro-Acupuncture on Anovulation in Women with Polycystic Ovary Syndrome," *Acta Obstetricia et Gynecologica Scandinavica* 79, no. 3 (March 2000): 180–188.

25. B. Y. Chen, "Acupuncture Normalizes Dysfunction of Hypothalamic-Pituitary-Ovarian Axis," *Acupuncture and Electrotherapeutics Research* 22, no. 2 (1997): 97–108.

26. E. Stener-Victorin, "Reduction of Blood Flow Impedance in the Uterine Arteries of Infertile Women with Electro-Acupuncture," *Human Reproduction* 11, no. 6 (June 1996): 1314–1317. Published in Oxford, England.

27. S. Siterman, et al., "Effect of Acupuncture on Sperm Parameters of Males Suffering from Subfertility Related to Low Sperm Quality," *Archives of Andrology* 39, no. 2 (September–October 1997): 155–161.

28. R. Riegler, et al., "Correlation of Psychological Changes and Spermiogram Improvements Following Acupuncture," *Der Urologe* 23, no. 6, series A (November 1984): 329–333.

29. Standing Committee on the Scientific Evaluation of Dietary Reference Intakes, Food and Nutrition Board *Dietary Reference Intakes for Vitamin C, Vitamin E, Selenium, and Carotenoids* (National Academies Press, 2000).

30. L. K. Roth and H. S. Taylor, "Risks of Smoking to Reproductive Health: Assessment of Women's Knowledge," *American Journal of Obstetrics and Gynecology* 184, no. 5 (April 2001): 934–939.

31. M. G. Hull, "Delayed Conception and Active and Passive Smoking: The Avon Longitudinal Study of Pregnancy and Childhood Study Team," *Fertility and Sterility* 74, no. 4 (October 2000): 725–733.

32. R. B. Ness, "Cocaine and Tobacco Use and the Risk of Spontaneous Abortion," *New England Journal of Medicine* 340, no. 5 (February 4, 1999): 333–339.

33. M. Saraiya, et al., "Cigarette Smoking as a Risk Factor for Ectopic Pregnancy," *American Journal of Obstetrics and Gynecology* 178, no. 3 (March 1998): 493–498.

34. F. S. Facchini, "Insulin Resistance and Cigarette Smoking," *Lancet* 339, no. 8802 (May 9, 1992): 1128–1130.

35. Hajek, et al., "Randomized Comparative Trial of Nicotine Polacrilex, a Transdermal Patch, Nasal Spray, and an Inhaler," *Archives of Internal Medicine* 159, no. 17 (July 2000): 2033–2038.

36. J. Hughes, et al., "Antidepressants for Smoking Cessation," *Cochrane Database of Systematic Reviews* no. 4 (October 18, 2004): CD000031. Online.

37. P. B. Gold, et al., "Naturalistic, Self-Assignment Comparative Trial of Bupropion SR, a Nicotine Patch, or Both for Smoking Cessation Treatment in Primary Care," *American Journal on Addictions* 11, no. 4 (Fall 2002): 315–331.

38. D. D. Baird, et al., "Vaginal Douching and Reduced Fertility," *American Journal of Public Health* 86, no. 6 (June 1996): 844–850.

39. W. H. Chow, et al., "Vaginal Douching as a Potential Risk Factor for Tubal Ectopic Pregnancy," *American Journal of Obstetrics and Gynecology* 153, no. 7 (December 1, 1985): 727–729.

Chapter 8

1. T. Nordenberg, "Overcoming Infertility," *FDA Consumer* (January–February 1997).

Chapter 9

1. "Diet and Exercise Dramatically Delay Type 2 Diabetes: Diabetes Medication Metformin Also Effective," National Institute of Diabetes & Digestive & Kidney Diseases (2001).

2. C. Diez-Sanchez, et al., "Mitochondria from Ejaculated Human Spermatozoa Do Not Synthesize Proteins," *FEBS [Federation of European Biochemical Sciences] Letters* 553, nos. 1–2 (October 9, 2003): 205–208.

3. R. Beloosesky, et al., "Induction of Polycystic Ovary by Testosterone in Immature Female Rats: Modulation of Apoptosis and Attenuation of Glucose/Insulin Ratio," *International Journal of Molecular Medicine* 14, no. 2 (August 2004): 207–215.

4. G. M. Prelevic, et al., "Inhibitory Effect of Sandostatin on Secretion of Luteinizing Hormone and Ovarian Steroids in Polycystic Ovary Syndrome," *Lancet* 336, no. 8720 (October 13, 1990): 900–903.

5. P. O. Dale, et al., "The Impact of Insulin Resistance on the Outcome of Ovulation Induction with Low-Dose Follicle Stimulating Hormone in Women with Polycystic Ovary Syndrome," *Human Reproduction* 13, no. 3 (March 1998): 567–570. Published in Oxford, England.

6. M. J. Heard, et al., "Pregnancies Following Use of Metformin for Ovulation Induction in Patients with Polycystic Ovary Syndrome," *Fertility and Sterility* 77, no. 4 (April 2002): 669–773.

7. A. M. Saleh and H. S. Khalil, "Review of Nonsurgical and Surgical Treatment and the Role of Insulin Sensitizing Agents in the Management of Infer-

tile Women with Polycystic Ovary Syndrome," *Acta Obstetricia et Gynecologica Scandinavica* 83, no. 7 (July 2004): 614–621.

8. I. Hasegawa, et al., "Effect of Troglitazone on Endocrine and Ovulatory Performance in Women with Insulin Resistance–Related Polycystic Ovary Syndrome," *Fertility and Sterility* 71, no. 2 (February 1999): 323–327.

9. M. Amin, et al., "Minireview: Up-Date Management of Non Responder to Clomiphene Citrate in Polycystic Ovary Syndrome," *Kobe Journal of Medical Science* 49, nos. 3–4 (2003): 59–73.

10. A. M. Clark, et al., "Weight Loss in Obese Infertile Women Results in Improvement in Reproductive Outcome for All Forms of Fertility Treatment," *European Society for Human Reproduction and Embryology* 13, no. 6 (June 1998): 1502–1505.

11. Ibid.

12. M. Pinget, et al., "Infertility and Carbohydrate Metabolism: A Study of 93 Cases," *Semaine des Hopitaux* 58, no. 4 (January 28, 1982): 209–212.

13. A. M. Clark, et al., op. cit.

14. P. M. Piatti, et al., "Hypocaloric High-Protein Diet Improves Glucose Oxidation and Spares Lean Body Mass: Comparison to Hypocaloric High-Carbohydrate Diet," *Metabolism* 43, no. 12 (December 1994): 1481–1487.

15. A. Golay, et al., "Weight-Loss with Low or High Carbohydrate Diet?" *International Journal of Obesity and Related Metabolic Disorders* 20, no. 12 (December 1996): 1067–1072.

16. P. A. Torjesen, et al., "Lifestyle Changes May Reverse Development of the Insulin Resistance Syndrome: The Oslo Diet and Exercise Study—A randomized trial," *Diabetes Care* 20, no. 1 (January 1997): 26–31.

17. S. Colagiuri and J. Brand-Miller, "The 'Carnivore Connection'—Evolutionary Aspects of Insulin Resistance," *European Journal of Clinical Nutrition* 56, suppl. 1 (March 2002): S30–S35.

18. Ibid.

19. L. B. Craig, et al., "Increased Prevalence of Insulin Resistance in Women with a History of Recurrent Pregnancy Loss," *Fertility and Sterility* 78, no. 3 (September 2002): 487–490.

Chapter 10

1. G. Peluso, et al., "Cancer and Anticancer Therapy-Induced Modifications on Metabolism Mediated by Carnitine System," *Journal of Cellular Physiology* 182, no. 3 (March 2000): 339–350.

2. B. Gurbuz, et al., "Relationship between Semen Quality and Seminal Plasma Total Carnitine in Infertile Men," *Journal of Obstetrics and Gynæcology* 23, no. 6 (November 2003): 653–656.

3. M. Costa, et al., "L-Carnitine in Idiopathic Asthenozoospermia: A Multi-center Study—Italian Study Group on Carnitine and Male Infertility," *Andrologia* 26, no. 3 (May–June 1994): 155–159. See also E. Vicari, et al., "Antioxidant Treatment with Carnitines Is Effective in Infertile Patients with Prostatovesiculoepididymitis and Elevated Seminal Leukocyte Concentrations After Treatment with Nonsteroidal Anti-Inflammatory Compounds," *Fertility and Sterility* 78, no. 6 (December 2002) 1203–1208.

4. E. Vicari, et al., "Effects of Treatment with Carnitines in Infertile Patients with Prostato-Vesiculo-Epididymitis," *Human Reproduction* 16, no. 11 (November 2001): 2338–2342. Published in Oxford, England.

5. M. Yamamoto, et al., "New Treatment of Idiopathic Severe Oligozoospermia with Mast Cell Blocker: Results of a Single-Blind Study," *Fertility and Sterility* 64, no. 6 (December 1995): 1221–1223.

6. H. Hibi, et al., "The Treatment with Tranilast, a Mast Cell Blocker, for Idiopathic Oligozoospermia," *Archives of Andrology* 47, no. 2 (April–June 2001): 107–111.

7. S. Cayan, D. D. Apa, and E. Akbay, "Effect of Fexofenadine, a Mast Cell Blocker, in Infertile Men with Significantly Increased Testicular Mast Cells," *Asian Journal of Andrology* 4, no. 4 (December 2002): 291–294.

8. S. Matsuki, et al., "The Use of Ebastine, a Mast Cell Blocker, for Treatment of Oligozoospermia," *Archives of Andrology* 44, no. 2 (March–April 2000): 129–132.

9. A. Mancini, et al., "Coenzyme Q10 Concentrations in Normal and Pathological Human Seminal Fluid," *Journal of Andrology* 15, no. 6 (November–December 1994): 591–594.

10. A. Mancini, et al., "Relationship between Sperm Cell Ubiquinone and Seminal Parameters in Subjects with and without Varicocele," *Andrologia* 30, no. 1 (February–March 1998): 1–4.

11. G. Balercia, et al., "Coenzyme Q10 Levels in Idiopathic and Varicocele-Associated Asthenozoospermia," *Andrologia* 34, no. 2 (April 2002): 107–111.

12. G. Balercia, et al., "Coenzyme Q(10) Supplementation in Infertile Men with Idiopathic Asthenozoospermia: An Open, Uncontrolled Pilot Study," *Fertility and Sterility* 81, no. 1 (January 2004): 93–98.

13. D. Robak-Cholubek, et al., "Zinc Levels in Seminal Plasma and Sperm Density," *Ginekologia Polska* 69, no. 6 (June 1998): 490–493.

14. A. E. Omu, et al., "Treatment of Asthenozoospermia with Zinc Sulphate: Andrological, Immunological, and Obstetric Outcome," *European Journal of Obstetrics, Gynecology, and Reproductive Biology* 72, no. 2 (August 1998): 179–184.

15. P. Palan and R. Naz, "Changes in Various Antioxidant Levels in Human Seminal Plasma Related to Immunoinfertility," *Archives of Andrology* 36, no. 2 (March–April 1996): 139–143.

16. N. P. Gupta and R. Kumar, "Lycopene Therapy in Idiopathic Male Infertility—A Preliminary Report," *International Urology and Nephrology* 34, no. 3 (2002): 369–372.

17. National Institute for Occupational Safety and Health, 1997.

18. "The Effects of Workplace Hazards on Male Reproductive Health," (National Institute for Occupational Safety and Health, 1997).

19. M. De Rosa, et al., "Traffic Pollutants Affect Fertility in Men," *Human Reproduction* 18, no. 5 (May 2003): 1055–1061. Published in Oxford, England.

20. J. C. Hansen, and Y. Deguchi, "Selenium and Fertility in Animals and Man—A Review," *Acta Veterinaria Scandinavica* 37, no. 1 (1996): 19–30.

21. R. Kunzle, et al., "Semen Quality of Male Smokers and Nonsmokers in Infertile Couples," *Fertility and Sterility* 72, no. 2 (February 2003): 287–291.

22. S. Sepaniak, et al., "Negative Impact of Cigarette Smoking on Male Fertility: From Spermatozoa to the Offspring," *Journal de Gynecologie, Obstetrique,*

et Biologie de la Reproduction 33, no. 5 (September 2004): 384–390. Published in Paris.

23. S. A. Venners, et al., "Paternal Smoking and Pregnancy Loss: A Prospective Study Using a Biomarker of Pregnancy," *American Journal of Epidemiology* 159, no. 10 (May 15, 2004): 993–1001.

24. M. B. Bracken, et al., "Association of Cocaine Use with Sperm Concentration, Motility, and Morphology," *Fertility and Sterility* 53, no. 2 (February 1990): 315–322.

25. N. P. Boyadjiev, et al., "Reversible Hypogonadism and Azoospermia as a Result of Anabolic-Androgenic Steroid Use in a Bodybuilder with Personality Disorder: A Case Report," *Journal of Sports Medicine and Physical Fitness* 40, no. 3 (September 2000): 271–274.

26. M. R. Gazvani, et al., "Conservative Management of Azoospermia Following Steroid Abuse," *Human Reproduction* 12, no. 8 (August 1997): 1706–1708. Published in Oxford, England.

Chapter 11

1. J. T. France, et al., "A Prospective Study of the Preselection of the Sex of Offspring by Timing Intercourse Relative to Ovulation," *Fertility and Sterility* 41, no. 6 (June 1984): 894–900.

2. R. H. Gray, "Natural Family Planning and Sex Selection: Fact or Fiction?" *American Journal of Obstetrics and Gynecology* 165, no. 6, part 2 (December 1991): 1982–1984.

3. C. S. Griffith and D. A. Grimes, "The Validity of the Postcoital Test," *American Journal of Obstetrics and Gynecology* 162, no. 3 (March 1990): 615–620.

4. R. Munkelwitz and B. R. Gilbert, "Are Boxer Shorts Really Better? A Critical Analysis of the Role of Underwear Type in Male Subfertility," *Journal of Urology* 160, no. 4 (October 1998): 1329–1333.

5. M. L. Hannuksela and S. Ellahham, "Benefits and Risks of Sauna Bathing," *American Journal of Medicine* 110, no. 2 (February 1, 2001): 118–126.

6. F. Sommer, et al., "Impotence and Genital Numbness in Cyclists," *International Journal of Sports Medicine* 22, no. 6 (August 2001): 410–413.

7. A. Lucia, et al., "Reproductive Function in Male Endurance Athletes: Sperm Analysis and Hormonal Profile," *Journal of Applied Physiology* 81, no. 6 (December 1996): 2627–2636.

8. Y. Gebreegziabher, et al., "Sperm Characteristics of Endurance Trained Cyclists," *International Journal of Sports Medicine* 25, no. 4 (May 2004): 247–251.

9. W. H. Kutteh, et al., "Vaginal Lubricants for the Infertile Couple: Effect on Sperm Activity," *International Journal of Fertility and Menopausal Studies* 41, no. 4 (July–August 1996): 400–404.

Chapter 12

1. Institute of Medicine.

2. Rooney and Schauberger, "Excess Pregnancy Weight Gain and Long-Term Obesity: One Decade Later," *Obstetrics and Gynecology* 100, no. 2 (August 2002): 245–252.

3. Olson and Strawderman, "Modifiable, Behavioral Factors in a Biopsychosocial Model Predict Inadequate and Excessive Gestational Weight Gain," *Journal of the American Dietetic Association* 103: 48 (2003).

4. A. F. Castoldi, et al., "Neurotoxicity and Molecular Effects of Methylmercury," *Brain Research Bulletin* 55, no. 2 (May 15, 2001): 197–203.

5. J. A. Bakerink, et al., "Multiple Organ Failure After Ingestion of Pennyroyal Oil from Herbal Tea in Two Infants," *Pediatrics* 98, no. 5 (November 1996): 944–947.

6. American College of Obstetricians and Gynecologists Committee Opinion no. 267 (2002).

7. J. F. Clapp III, et al., "Beginning Regular Exercise in Early Pregnancy: Effect on Fetoplacental Growth," *American Journal of Obstetrics and Gynecology* 183, no. 6 (December 2000): 1484–1488.

8. A. Jonasson, et al., "Testing and Training of the Pelvic Floor Muscles After Childbirth," *Acta Obstetricia et Gynecologica Scandinavica* 68, no. 4 (1989): 301–304.

Bibliography

Achard, C., and J. Thiers. "Le virilisme pilaire et son association à l'insuffisance glycolytique (diabète des femmes à barb)." *Bulletin de l'Académie Nationale de Médecine* 86 (1921): 51–64.

Agatston, S. *The South Beach Diet: The Delicious, Doctor-Designed, Foolproof Plan for Fast and Healthy Weight Loss.* Ephrata, PA: Rodale, 2003.

Atkins, R. C. *Dr. Atkins' New Diet Revolution.* 3rd ed. New York: Evans, 2002.

Bates, G., and M. S. Whitworth. "Effects of Body Weight Reduction on Plasma Androgens in Obese, Infertile Women." *Fertility and Sterility* 38 (1982): 406–409.

Broussard, B. A., E. Brzezinski, N. Cooper, et al. "The First Step in Meal Planning." American Diabetes Association and American Dietetic Association, 1995. (Patient instruction pamphlet.)

Burghen, G. A., J. R. Givens, and A. E. Kitabchi. "Correlation of Hyperandrogenism with Hyperinsulinism in Polycystic Ovarian Disease." *Journal of Clinical Endocrinology and Metabolism* 50 (1980): 113–116.

Carey, D. G., A. B. Jenkins, L. V. Campbell, et al. "Abdominal Fat and Insulin Resistance in Normal and Overweight Women: Direct Measurements Reveal a Strong Relationship in Subjects at Both Low and High Risk of NIDDM." *Diabetes* 45 (1996): 633–638.

Clark, A. M., B. Thornley, L. Tomlinson, et al. "Weight Loss in Obese Infertile Women Results in Improvement in Reproductive Outcome for All Forms of Fertility Treatment." *Human Reproduction* 13 (1998): 1502–1505.

Cline, G. W., K. F. Petersen, M. Shen, et al. "Impaired Glucose Transport as a Cause of Decreased Insulin-Stimulated Muscle Glycogen Synthesis in Type 2 Diabetes." *New England Journal of Medicine* 341 (1999): 240–245.

Coulston, A. M., G. C. Liu, and G. M. Reaven. "Plasma, Glucose, Insulin, and Lipid Responses to High-Carbohydrate, Low-Fat Diets in Normal Humans." *Metabolism* 32 (1983): 52–56.

Crave, J., S. Fimbel, H. Lejeune, et al. "Effects of Diet and Metformin Administration on Sex Hormone–Binding Globulin, Androgens, and Insulin in Hirsute and Obese Women." *Journal of Clinical Endocrinology and Metabolism* 80 (1995): 2057–2062.

Dale, P. O., T. Tanbo, E. Huag, and T. Abyholm. "The Impact of Insulin Resistance on the Outcome of Ovulation Induction with Low-Dose Follicle Stimulating Hormone in Women with Polycystic Ovary Syndrome." *Human Reproduction* 13 (1998): 567–570.

Dunaif, A. "Insulin Resistance and the Polycystic Ovary Syndrome: Mechanism and Implications for Pathogenesis." *Endo Reviews* 18, no. 6 (1997): 774–800.

———, M. Graf, J. Mandeli, et al. "Characterization of Groups of Hyperandrogenic Women with Acanthosis Nigricans, Impaired Glucose Tolerance, and/or Hyperinsulinemia." *Journal of Clinical Endocrinology and Metabolism* 65 (1987): 499–507.

———, K. R. Segal, W. Futtereweit, and A. Drobrjansky. "Profound Peripheral Insulin Resistance, Independent of Obesity, in Polycystic Ovary Syndrome." *Diabetes* 38 (1989): 1165–1174.

Golay, A., C. Eigenheer, Y. Morel, et al. "Weight-Loss with Low or High Carbohydrate Diet?" *International Journal of Obesity and Related Metabolic Disorders* 20 (1996): 1067–1072.

Guzick, D. S. "Polycystic Ovary Syndrome: Symptomatology, Pathophysiology, and Epidemiology." *American Journal of Obstetrics and Gynecology* 179 (1998): S89–S92.

———, R. Wing, D. Smith, and S. L. Berga. "Endocrine Consequences of Weight Loss in Obese, Hyperandrogenic, Anovulatory women." *Fertility and Sterility* 61 (1994): 598–604.

Hasegawa, I., H. Murakawa, M. Suzuki, et al. "Effect of Troglitazone on Endocrine and Ovulatory Performance in Women with Insulin Resistance— Related Polycystic Ovary Syndrome." *Fertility and Sterility* 71 (1999): 323–327.

Heavin, G., and C. Colman. *Curves: Permanent Results Without Permanent Dieting.* New York: Putnam, 2003.

Huber-Buchholz, M. M., D. G. P. Carey, and R. J. Norman. "Restoration of Reproductive Potential by Lifestyle Modification in Obese Polycystic

Ovary Syndrome: Role of Insulin Sensitivity and Luteinizing Hormone." *Journal of Clinical Endocrinology and Metabolism* 84 (1999): 1470–1474.

Kaczmarski, R. J., K. M. Flegal, S. M. Comptede, and C. L. Johnson. "Increasing Prevalence of Overweight Among U.S. Adults." *Journal of the American Medical Association* 272 (1994): 205–239.

Legro, R. S., D. T. Finegood, and A. Dunaif. "A Fasting Glucose to Insulin Ratio Is a Useful Measure of Insulin Sensitivity in Women with Polycystic Ovary Syndrome." *Journal of Clinical Endocrinology and Metabolism* 183 (1998): 2694–2699.

Modan, M., M. I. Harris, and H. Halkin. "Evaluation of WHO and NDDG Criteria for Impaired Glucose Tolerance: Results from Two National Samples." *Diabetes* 38 (1989): 1630–1635.

Nestle, M. *Food Politics*. Berkeley: University of California Press, 2003.

Pasquali, R., F. Casimirri, and V. Vicennati. "Weight Control and Its Beneficial Effect on Fertility in Women with Obesity and Polycystic Ovary Syndrome." *Human Reproduction* 12S (1997): 82–87.

Piatti, P. M., F. Monti, I. Fermo, et al. "Hypocaloric High-Protein Diet Improves Glucose Oxidation and Spares Lean Body Mass: Comparison to Hypocaloric High-Carbohydrate Diet." *Metabolism* 43 (1994): 1481–1487.

Pinget, M., P. Dufour, R. Gandar, et al. "[Infertility and Carbohydrate Metabolism. A Study of 93 Cases.]" *Semaine des Hôpitaux* 58 (1982): 209–212. (In French.)

Reindollar, R. H., M. Novak, S. P. T. Tho, and P. G. McDonough. "Adult-Onset Amenorrhea: A Study of 262 Patients." *American Journal of Obstetrics and Gynecology* 155 (1986): 531–543.

Sadur, C. N., and R. H. Eckel. "Insulin Stimulation of Adipose Tissue Lipoprotein Lipase." *Journal of Clinical Investigation* 69 (1982): 1119–1123.

Sears, B., and B. Lawren. *Enter the Zone: A Dietary Road Map*. New York: HarperCollins, 1995.

Shepherd, P. R., and B. B. Kahn. "Glucose Transporters and Insulin Action: Implications for Insulin Resistance and Diabetes Mellitus." *New England Journal of Medicine* 341 (1999): 248–256.

Swisklocki, A. M., Y. D. Chen, M. A. Golay, et al. "Insulin Suppression of Plasma-Free Fatty Acid Concentration in Normal Individuals or Patients with Type 2 (Non-Insulin-Dependent) Diabetes." *Diabetologia* 30 (1987): 622–626.

Torjesen, P. A., K. I. Birkeland, S. A. Anderssen, et al. "Lifestyle Changes May Reverse Development of the Insulin Resistance Syndrome: The Oslo Diet and Exercise Study—A Randomized Trial." *Diabetes Care* 20 (1997): 26–31.

Ulene, A. *The NutriBase Complete Book of Food Counts.* New York: Avery, 1996.

Wolever, T. M. S. "Relationship between Dietary Fiber Content and Composition in Foods and the Glycemic Index." *American Journal of Clinical Nutrition* 51 (1990): 72–75.

———, D. J. A. Jenkins, A. A. Jenkins, and R. G. Josse. "The Glycemic Index: Methodology and Clinical Implications." *American Journal of Clinical Nutrition* 54 (1991): 846–854.

Zawedzki, J. K., and A. Dunaif. "Diagnostic Criteria for Polycystic Ovary Syndrome: Toward a Rational Approach." In *Polycystic Ovary Syndrome,* edited by A. Dunaif, J. R. Givens, F. P. Haseltine, and G. R. Merriam. Boston: Blackwell Scientific, 1992, pp. 377–384.

Zhang, L., H. Rodriguez, S. Ohno, and W. L. Miller. "Serine Phosphorylation of Human P450c17 Increases 17,20 Lyase Activity: Implications for Adrenarche and the Polycystic Ovary Syndrome." *Proceedings of the National Academy of Sciences of the United States* 92 (1995): 10619–10623.

Acknowledgments

Bouquets of gratitude go out to all the people who helped bring this fertility nutrition and fitness program to print. Night-blooming jasmine goes to our nocturnal word wizard, Jenna Glatzer, who brought depth, experience, and laughter to this project. No one could dream of a better contributing writer. Roses go to Joëlle Delbourgo, our agent, and Nancy Hancock, our editor. Their professionalism, knowledge, and insight made this journey possible. A spring bouquet goes out to Sarah Peach, Nancy's assistant, whose involvement in this project always provided a breath of fresh air.

Carolina bluebells go to Marc Fritz, M.D.; Bruce Lessey, M.D., Ph.D; William Meyer, M.D.; Ania Kowalik, M.D.; Stan Beyler, Ph.D.; Rebecca Usadi, M.D.; Ringland Murray, M.D.; Pamela Richey M.S.; Eileen Petersen, R.N.; Mary Gruenwald, R.N.; Carolyn Montgomery, R.N.; and Angela Shatley, R.N., who worked with Jeremy during his fellowship at UNC Chapel Hill. This foundation of knowledge and support created the ideal environment to fine-tune this program.

A vast mixed bouquet goes to Jeremy's many patients who were willing to go beyond the pill-popping mentality and work on their own lifestyle in an effort to conceive. We commend their hard work and dedication to this program. Their feedback has been invaluable. A fiesta of flowers goes to our friends and family: the Clarks, the Stovalls, the Butchers, the Rhoads, the Diedrichs, the Nowaks, and the

Grolls provided us with incredible support during the conception of this program. They watched our children, listened to our ideas, taste tested our recipes, and were terrific cheerleaders during this crazy time.

Sweet peas go out to our children: Libby, Michael, and Lainey, who sacrificed the most while we worked on this dream of ours; you continue to fill our lives with fun and inspiration. Pansies go out to the many more people who have added points of light to this process. And most important, daffodils to all the children who may be conceived through the use of the information found in this book.

Index

About the Authors

DR. JEREMY GROLL is a reproductive endocrinologist, specializing in the treatment of infertile couples. As a Junior Fellow of the Society for Reproductive Endocrinology and Infertility (SREI), Jeremy is a member of one of the most exclusive sub-specialty organizations in all of medicine. He recently finished his OB/GYN sub-specialty fellowship training at the University of North Carolina, Chapel Hill. His educational background also includes an undergraduate degree from Notre Dame, a medical school degree from Wayne State University in Detroit, Michigan, and the completion of his internship and residency at Wilford Hall Medical Center at Lackland Air Force Base in Texas.

Jeremy is a recipient of a research grant from the Surgeon General's Office to study the role of diet in fertility. He was recently named the recipient of the American Society for Reproductive Medicine's (ASRM) Fellow Research Prize Paper and of the American College of Obstetrics and Gynecology's (ACOG) Founder's Award, both national awards for basic science research.

LORIE GROLL juggles caring for their three children, managing Delphinos Enterprises (the Grolls' Internet-based health and nutrition business), and finishing her master's in education at the University of North Carolina, Chapel Hill. With a mother who was a nutritionist, Lorie grew up with a strong understanding of the importance of diet and food preparation. Cooking has been a passion for Lorie since she could pull a chair up to reach the counter as a child. She has always loved to experiment in the kitchen, though her recipes have come a long way since her walnut cakes with turquoise frosting. Creating recipes for this program that are delicious and balanced has been a delightful challenge. Lorie's undergraduate degree in English from the Colorado College provided the foundation for her former career as a freelance technical writer for nonprofit organizations, high-tech companies, and drug development firms. She has enjoyed using her writing and culinary skills to help Jeremy serve his patients.